Urhobo Traditional Medicine

Urhobo Traditional Medicine

John Oroshẹjẹdẹ Ubrurhe

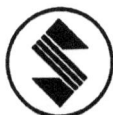

Spectrum Books Limited
Ibadan
Abuja • Benin City • Lagos • Owerri

Spectrum titles can be purchased on line at
www.spectrumbooksonline.com

Published by:
Spectrum Books Limited
Spectrum House
Ring Road
PMB 5612
Ibadan, Nigeria.
e-mail: *admin1@spectrumbooksonline.com*

in association with
Safari Books (Export) Limited
1st Floor
17 Bond Street
St Helier
Jersey JE2 3NP
Channel Islands
United Kingdom

Europe and USA Distributor
African Books Collective Ltd.
The Jam Factory
27, Park End Street
Oxford OX1, 1HU, UK

First published, 2001 by Oputoru Books
This edition is published by Spectrum Books Ltd, 2003

ISBN: 978-029-406-6

Printed by Sam-Adex Printers, Felele Rab, Ibadan

DEDICATION

To my wife, **Esther Ufuoma,**
for her love and encouragement in the family.

CONTENTS

FOREWORD

Health is essential to life as a signal of the sanctity which hedges it. Health is about wholeness and the maintenance of the balance in existence — balance in cosmic order, in the relationship between humans and other inhabitants of the psychic environment, balance in social and human relationship with the supernatural. Health has psychic, social and religious dimensions and health care practices seek to nurture, preserve, restore and enhance wholeness. Health is an antidote to brokenness and medicine is the agency. Ritual agents diagnose, prescribe and apply medicine to combat various types of brokenness. Some are internally induced and others come through external sources such as witchcraft, sorcery, ecological pollution and war.

Oroshẹjẹdẹ John Ubrurhe's *Urhobo Traditional Medicine* has the distinction of using a major ethnic group as an in-depth case study to explore Urhobo Medicine; definition, taxonomy, causality and therapy. Such details of Urhobo Pharmacognosy and therapeutics will enable a comparative perspective. Of major significance is the specific role of religion. It is argued that religion proffers a certain interpretation for the meaning of life. It provides an explanation, prediction and control of space-time events. It enhances various means of sustaining life. For instance, it is the spiritual dimension which gives potency to the herbs. Otherwise, leaves are merely leaves. But this raises the question about the relationship between rituals and efficacy. Without religious rituals, will herbs treated within laboratories, perform efficaciously?

The significance of this question comes from two angles. Some people are worried that western medicine is chemical-based with injurious side effects, that organic perception of life links humans to nature for mutual sustenance, that it is healthier to return to the old indigenous orders of healing. Secondly, the quest for an alternative medicine is now in vogue and an aspect of government policy. Some claim that it is cheaper, others emphasise the environmental dimension. John's work is essential in building the fundamental basis for research and policy. It is an innovative work as an aspect of cultural construction on Urhobo people. One reads this work with much satisfaction and hopes that such a candle is not hidden under a bushel.

Professor Ogbu U. Kalu
Centre for the Study of World Religions
Harvard University

xi

PREFACE

Life is the greatest gift from the Creator, God, and by extrapolation it belongs to Him. In all the creation mythologies, be they traditional or biblical, no creature apart from man has an intimate relationship with *Oghene*, the Supreme Being and Creator. Perhaps for illustrative purpose, the biblical account demonstrates immutably a premeditated conception about man's creation. God says, "Let us make man in our image, after our likeness; and let them have dominion over the fish of the sea, and over the birds of the air, and over the cattle, and over all the earth, and over every creeping thing that creeps upon the earth" (Gen. 1:26). (Gen. 2:7) portrays the personal involvement of the Creator in the formation of man this way: "Then the Lord God formed man out of dust from the ground, and breathed into his nostrils the breath of life; and man became a living being." While in the creation of other phenomena in the universe, the Creator only verbalized his intention but in the creation of man, the Creator physically participated.

Most African myths of creation do not differ radically from that of the Hebrews. In Africa, man's soul, the spark of the Creator, is believed to be indestructible. One such story that readily springs to mind is the popular Yoruba creation myth which clearly depicts the different roles performed by Olodumare and Orisanla, the archdivinity.

This singular position which man occupies in the cosmos as the major phenomenon that would give meaning to the universe made *Oghene* endow man with the ability to feed on and take control over all other creatures for his betterment. By the same token, the central and precarious position of man was not unknown to *Oghene*. Hence life diminutive agents of diseases, discomfort and affliction were catered for by the provision of means of counteracting them. Thus the growth and development of medical system to preserve, cure, restore and enhance life in all its ramifications of wholeness are traceable to *Oghene*.

In all aggregates of humans and in all cultures, there is a medical system that caters for the health of the group. This distinct medical system is often designated as traditional medicine - medicine as practised in the earliest times without external accoutrement and tinge of science and technology. Traditional Medicine in this context was, and is, present among all the peoples of the world. Thus Urhobo medicine, which is the focus of this work, is the medical system as practised by the Urhobo progenitors and later handed down to their progeny.

This work was necessitated firstly by the ageing and death of the custodians and practitioners of the Urhobo medical system: for without proper documentation, this aspect of Urhobo cultural heritage would be lost. Consequently, the work is aimed at providing an Urhobo pharmacopoeia to facilitate further pharmacological analysis of Urhobo traditional medicines. Secondly, the Urhobo Christians, Moslems and elites have been so brainwashed that they view the medical system as primitive, inefficacious and its practice is termed paganism. Thirdly, there is a clarion call to drift from synthetic medicine to galenical and medicinal plant treatment.

The work attempts at examining the Urhobo worldview as it relates to the practice of medicine, investigating the use of incantations and rituals in both Urhobo and western medical systems, examining people's claim to its efficacy or not, providing examples of medicinal plants and the diseases they cure and providing a balanced argument that Urhobo medicine, like its western counterpart, is provided by God to cater for the diminutive agents of life. Ultimately, this will lead to the pharmacological analysis of Urhobo medicine since effective scientific analysis cannot occur if the traditional pharmacological utility of the medicinal plants is not provided. This work is, therefore, an attempt to provide information on Urhobo medicine. It is hoped that the knowledge gained from this work will be an immense contribution to a global research into traditional medicinal plants. It will, no doubt, aid the upgrading of the Urhobo health delivery system.

In this work, "Afrel" the acronym of African Traditional Religion will be used. The work is divided into five chapters.

Chapter One introduces the reader to African traditional medicine. The definitions of important terms like tradition, medicine, traditional medicine, magic and sorcery and its practitioners and campaign of vilification against traditional medicine are also investigated.

A people's understanding of the world around them (worldview) determines their practice of medicine; to understand Urhobo medicine, therefore, the worldview approach has been chosen.

Chapter Two deals with this and the comparison of the Urhobo and Western Cosmologies in an attempt to highlight their similarities and differences. The chapter also deals with taxonomy which is sub-divided into A, B and C. Taxonomy A deals with disease typology; Taxonomy B examines therapeutic modalities and Taxonomy C focuses on different categories of medicine, magic, sorcery and witchcraft.

Diagnosis and treatment are the focus of *Chapter Three*. The diagnosis and treatment of different diseases are discussed. The functions of incantations and rituals in Urhobo medical system are also examined. Attempt is also made at a comparative study of ritual and efficacy in both Urhobo and

Western medical systems. Examples of some diseases and their cure and prevention are given in this chapter. To make the medicines meaningful to the people in Urhobo culture areas, names of herbs in the four culture areas have been given.

Chapter Four is the evaluation of Urhobo medicine. It investigates the contributions of Urhobo medicine in barrenness in women, impotency in men, fractures and treatment of psychosocial and supernatural diseases. Like every other medical system, Urhobo medicine has defects. Some of its practitioners have been accused of claiming to be adepts in the treatment of all ailments, they are also accussed of secrecy, receipt of money before revealing medicine, overdosage and practising under insanitary conditions. These defects are thoroughly examined and proper recommendations made where necessary.

Chapter Five summarises the various arguments involved in the work. It argues that Urhobo medicine as a distinct medical system differs from its western counterparts in the use of incantations and rituals. Thus, although incantations and some rituals may be meaningless to the casual observer, they form an integral aspect of Urhobo medicine.

In conclusion, it must be emphasized that this work is seminal because it is the first attempt at providing Urhobo pharmacopoeia. By this work, the existing gap between Urhobo and other peoples, who have developed their pharmacopoeia, is bridged. Recommendations have been made here on how best to provide and conserve medicinal plants in Urhoboland. Urhobo Christians, elites and agnostics are urged to divest themselves of their negative attitudes consequent on the missionary and colonial agents' campaign of vilification against Urhobo medicine and its practitioners.

J. O. Ubrurhe
March 2001

ACKNOWLEDGEMENTS

At various stages of this work, a number of people were very useful to me. Their contributions are so immense that I remain grateful to them all. It is not possible to mention all their names, yet some names must be mentioned.

I remain deeply indebted to Professor Ogbu U. Kalu for his patience, encouragement and lifestyle which enable him to make every available space a classroom and office. Besides, he not only introduced me to scholarly works of eminent persons but also made available to me his relevant journals, articles and books. Professor, you are worthy of emulation.

I am aware of the different contributions that all the members of the academic staff of the Department of Religion, University of Nigeria, Nsukka, made towards the successful completion of this work. To the Head of Department, Rev. Fr. E. I. Ifesieh, I owe the enthusiasm to proceed to the Ph.D. work. He really spurred me to hard work in order to improve on my performance during my Master's programme. Rev. (Dr.) N. Onwu bailed me out of my difficulty when the way to the realization of my dream seemed blurred and uncertain. Dr. S. O. Onyeidu and Rev. Fr. (Dr.) O. A. Ekwunife encouraged and urged me to complete the work earlier than now. Thank you all for your encouragement.

My colleagues of the Department of Religious Studies, Delta State, University, Abraka assisted me in various ways. I owe Rev. Fr. L. A. Attah a debt of gratitude for his material, financial and moral assistance. Mr. E. F. Eghwubare deserves special attention and thanks. He took special interest in the work by reading through the manuscript and suggesting some corrections. Professor D. T. Adamo who recently took up appointment with the University also contributed immensely to the work. His foresightedness and advice have contributed a lot to my method of approach to sensitive issues.

Messrs. W. Onoriose, J. E. Denedo and F. Ekama's contributions are also worthy of note. During moments of frustration and disillusionment, discussions with these personages spurred and brightened me up. Mr. E. Idolor of the Department of Applied and Performing Arts and my Sandwich Programme student, Mr. G. O. Emesiri who acted as interpreters in the Okpe and Uvwie and Ethiope Culture areas; their contributions are noteworthy.

I am also indebted to Dr. J. O. Mume and Chief (Dr.) R. A. O. Uko, renowned traditional medical officers, whose works and interviews, have contributed in no small way to the success of this work. Chief (Dr.) R. A. O. Uko was the national Vice-President of Nigerian Herbal Practitioners while Professor Lambo was the Chairman.

I am grateful to my aged mother, Mrs. Ekpetuidi Ubrurhe, for being patient with me in my irregular payment of her monthly maintenance allowance. I owe what I am today to her and my brother, Mark Edafeadjeke, who trained me from Secondary Modern School up to the University level.

I extend my warmest regards to Mr. J. O. Ehiagwina for typing the original Ph.D thesis work. The book was originally typeset by Miss. Dorcas Benson of Oputoru Books. I thank her heartily for her expertise.

Many scholars whose works were relevant and useful have been duly acknowledged in the end notes, references and bibliography. The extent of the bibliography indicates my degree of indebtedness.

I am also grateful to the medicine men, diviners, priests and non-professionals whom I interviewed. I am particularly grateful to the non-professionals for divulging their medicines.

I wish to express my profound gratitude to the Delta State University for gratefully inheriting my shuttle leave from the defunct Bendel State University.

Finally, Egbe Ifie of the University of Ibadan who took interest in my Ph.D thesis and fondly asked me to revisit it for publication should accept my thanks.

J. O. Ubrurhe
Department of Religious Studies
Delta State University,
Abraka.

CHAPTER ONE

Understanding African Traditional Medicine

INTRODUCTION

The twenty-first century is witnessing serious efforts to discover the active principles in African medicinal plants. This urge has become more vigorous with the scientific findings that diseases are becoming more resistant to systematic medicines especially antibiotics. In the United States of America for instance, the number of days a patient is expected to stay in hospital for medical treatment has been increased by 3-5 days because of their induced side effects.[1] This, no doubt, has caused much concern to different world governments, especially those of the industrialized countries. This concern is manifest in the recent movement away from the use of synthetic medicine to galenical and the use of medicinal plants which form about 90% of the traditional medicine.

Secondly, the World Health Organization (WHO) by introducing the Health for All programme realized that the achievement of this objective could not be through orthodox medical practice only. WHO, therefore, encourages the use of all available medical systems, both orthodox and traditional. To this end, efforts are being made to provide enough data on traditional medicine so that intensive scientific research can be carried out on the constituents of medicinal plants. Kokwora[2] and Iwu[3] emphasize the need to update the data bank by carrying out further study on medicinal plants' chemical composition and their reactions upon the diseases in question.

Iwu, however, sees the inability to provide useful data on African medicine as a bane to its scientific study. As he observes: "Effective scientific reasoning depends first of all on access to evidence. Without a number of technical aids, the vastly greater part of our relevant evidence would still be hidden from us". Such scientific research will, no doubt, assist in the isolation of new and useful medicinal agents. For instance, *strophanthus* which is employed in traditional medicine for the cure of venereal diseases and heart troubles has been isolated and is today used pharmacologically as cardiotonic. In the same way, *digitalis* was used in Europe as a domestic medicine for external application until 1776 when Withering recognized and recommended its cardiotonic properties.[4]

1

The successful isolation of the active properties of *strophanthus* and *digitalis* and other such medicinal plants would have been impossible if the traditional utility was unknown. However, attempts are being made to investigate Nigerian medicinal plants especially among the Yoruba and Igbo, through the scholarly works of Iwu (1981), Ohiaeri (n.d) Ezeabasili (1977), among the Igbo; Sofola (1973), Dopamu (1977, 1978, 1983, 1985, 1987), Ayoade (1979), Prince (1966), Una Maclean (1971) and a host of others who have provided traditional useful information on some Yoruba medicinal plants. This has consequently led to the establishment of Department of Pharmacognosy in the Faculty of Pharmacy in some Nigerian Universities.

It is lamentable that while much has been achieved in the isolation of active principles from medicinal plants among the Yoruba and Igbo in Nigeria, nobody has attempted to provide any information on Urhobo traditional medicine which will, no doubt, act as a fillip for the take-off of an effective pharmacological study of Urhobo medicinal plants. In this regard, no meaningful study has been undertaken to provide the needed data for further pharmacological investigation. It is the aim of this work to provide such required data.

The examination of the available literature will form a base for theoretical framework for investigating Urhobo traditional medicine. The review will be executed under the following:

(i)   Provenance of medicine;

(ii)   Definition of traditional medicine, magic, and sorcery;

(iii) Early views about traditional medicine and its practitioners.

PROVENANCE OF MEDICINE

In all religious traditions, their mythologies depict that the Supreme Being, by whatever name He is known, is the Creator of man and the world suffused with all types of flora, fauna and other materials for consumption. In the Hebrew mythology, the omniscient God and King Unique was perhaps conscious of the multi-dimensional factors responsible for the diminution of health that He specifically directed man to eat all plants, fruits, animals and other consumable materials in the earth to counteract the effects of the various diminutive agents.

In the course of the consumption of these plants, fruits, animals and other materials, man discovered that some had therapeutic properties. The provenance of medicine is traceable to this process of trial and error experience. Iwu traces the origin of medicine to man's quest for food; an attempt which made him taste all edible materials. To him, the ancient man did not see any sharp distinction between food and medicine from a utilitarian viewpoint. He contends that of the many ancient *materia medica,* only very few toxic medicines were included and that most of the medicinal plants were used as food. Thus, their natural food contained many necessary and useful chemicals which helped in the maintenance of optimum health. As Brekhman puts it:

> In the search for food, ancient peoples tasted all that grows in the earth, that crawls and walks over it, that flies above it and lives in the waters... the plants, animals, birds, fishes and invertebrates. People noticed in this process that along with satiation, other sensations arise; different moods...and sometimes the cure of ailments[5]

Iwu also asserts that the various chemicals present in food determine and differentiate the various dietary habits of peoples from diverse parts of the world and the prevalence of certain diseases in specific ethnic or racial groups. However, Harley[6] differentiates man's experimental use of plant from animal's in the attempt to procure good therapeutics from the multifarious materials available. Smith[7] and Ayoade[8] go further to give the distinct characteristics of therapeutic plants which guided man in his trial and error. Alland (Jr.)[9] opines that it was through this means that people all over the world have developed different medical systems for preserving, restoring, enhancing life and means of achieving their life aspirations whenever life falls into a state of discomfort, disease and ill-health.

Mume[10] supports the argument that the origin of medicine is found in the trial and error method guided by man's three senses of sight, taste and touch. He further argues that this trial and error method must have made man taste some poisonous plants which must have led to the death of many people. Mume's point of view is conjectural. If man was guided by the three senses he has mentioned, he would not have eaten much of the medicinal trees to the extent that it could poison him. He would rather take little quantity at a time since man was also guided by his innate tendency of self-preservation.

Mume also attributes the origin of medicine to *juju* priests who burnt smelling substances of herbal material to produce sweet incense to appease the "gods of medicine". This, he argues, gave the priests the awareness that such sweet smelling plants could be used as curatives for some form of diseases. He further uses this point to substantiate the fact that *juju* priests were the medicine men of the people. He also observes that medicine must have originated from the kind gods of medicine and gods of war; a knowledge which was later transmitted from generation to generation.

The last source of the origin of medicine, Mume contends, is derived from man's observation and imitation of how the beasts treat themselves when they are unwell. He substantiates this concept with a traditional midwife who has efficacious herbal remedies for delivery from her observation of self-treatment by her nanny goat which was in labour. After taking the remedy, in less than five minutes, it was delivered of two kids. Later the midwife tried it on a pregnant woman during labour and she was easily and quickly delivered of a bouncing baby. Mume asserts that through these various methods of origin of medicine, all countries and tribes have their traditional medicine handed down to them by their forebears. He notes that these varied traditional medical systems have been improved upon from time to time to the stage of perfection.

Oguakwa [11] attributes the origin of medicine to early man's observation of the consistencies in the patterns and chains of natural phenomena. Consequently, man achieved how he could manipulate natural laws to his own advantages. He posits that this empirical acquisition of knowledge was later extended to plants and man discovered that some of them were useful as food, others were poisonous while man found another group of plants to possess medicinal properties. These discoveries, Oguakwa argues, were noted and this special knowledge was later transmitted to man's progeny.

Oguakwa defines a medicinal plant as "any plant which contains in any part of its organs substances that can be applied for therapeutic uses or substances that are precursors for chemopharmaceutical semisynthesis." These remedies in medical plants, Oguakwa contends, are provided by the Creator of the cosmos. Oguakwa's assertion supports the trial and error experience and the law of signature.

The theory of the law of signature according to Oliver [12] states that nature has provided a plant for every disease or for which part of the body each drug plant is to be used. This belief also existed in Europe in the Middle Ages and a classical example was the walnut which has the shape of the brain and was used for diseases affecting the brain. Similarly in West Africa, plants with white juice are used to increase milk production; those with big swollen fruits to increase fertility and commelina with its bright blue flower-like eyes is used for the treatment of eye problems.

Alland (Jr.) views the systematic development of medicine in every culture as emanating from the same experimental perspective. As he puts it:

> A system of medicine is produced by every culture. In medicine, a department of knowledge and practice dealing with disease and its treatment, man uses language of symbols when he observes, describes or thinks about the world of disease. The grouping of these observations, descriptions and thoughts leads to a certain conceptual orientation. [13]

This is also the attestation of Dopamu. [14] However, Nze [15] traces the source and the date of the practice of charm medicine to beyond the memory of man. Nze's statement implies that the source and practice of medicine are coeval with man. We may assent that the source of medicine is beyond man's memory because the *materia medica* were created by the Supreme Being but the practice of medicine which was started by man could not have been beyond the memory of man. We can rather say that the date of the practice of medicine is lost to man's memory.

Winterbottom [16] examines the progress of medicine. He observes that the origin of medicine has probably been the same in every culture, its progress towards perfection has been equally slow and gradual in all. Dopamu traces the origin of the knowledge of the different diseases and their cure in Africa to the curious attitude of Africans to know. Dopamu, therefore, remarks:

> It is the curiosity that leads them to their knowledge of phenomena, their observation of the behaviour of plants and animals, their expression of the mystery of the universe and their discovery of the therapeutic properties of natural objects generally. [17]

While accepting the view that the origin of medicine is traceable to trial and error experience, it must be noted that man who has the revelation of the Supreme Being must have been guided, to some extent, by his innate tendency of self-preservation and natural disposition. All men at the early stage of development were close to nature and the creator.

The origin of medicine is often traced to Africa, especially Egypt, the cradle of civilization. Winterbottom opines that the world is indebted for at least the rudiments of this art to the Africans no matter how despicable their knowledge of it may appear at present. [18] Iwu puts it succinctly that Egypt left the rest of the world behind in medical knowledge; that it is an accepted fact that the early Egyptians were Africans and therefore, much of the glory of the advances in modern medicine belongs rightly to Africa. He illustrates with how scholars were baffled by the complete interpenetration of magico-spiritual and "rational" elements of Egyptian medicine. [19] Sadly enough, African medical system has remained about the least developed. Various reasons have been advanced for the slow rate of improvement in African medical system. Winterbottom attributes this to the great pugnacity of the Africans to change customs which long usage rendered venerable. [20] Other scholars put the blame on the slave trade which slowed down the rate of scientific development in the continent.

Winterbottom's reason does not account adequately for the slow rate of progress in African medical system. Throughout world history, man has resisted innovations which ultimately displace already existing and well-established order. Nduka's [21] views change as inescapable aspect of human life. He asserts that these changes may occur in techniques, religious beliefs and practices, customs, economic and political organizations; changes in knowledge and, at a more rarefied level, conceptual systems. To Nduka, these are the stuff of human life throughout the world. He opines that it is part of human nature and of societies to resist change, especially those in positions of leadership, through age, inheritance, personal achievement and even through *coup d'etat*, that would upset the status quo. He went further to contend that they only entertain changes in so far as such changes are to their interest or the group to which they belong in the long or the short term. Even in the realm of medicine this was also true. Youngson who examined scientific revolution in Victorian medicine documents the stern opposition the innovations like the sterilization of the syringe, the anaesthesia chloroform and antisepsis experienced by the force of tradition. He argues that:

> New ideas in any sphere of life are often met with hostility is a well-known fact. Whatever is established is of proven usefulness, its limitations as well as its values are understood, it has the support of time, and perhaps also of famous and reputed names; on the other hand, what is new is yet untried. Moreover, new devices or new technologies or even new designs are likely to require the user to learn and to adapt, and learning and adaptation are not agreeable to everyone especially to those who are old enough to be set in their ways of thinking and doing.[22]

We may therefore turn to the other school of thought which blames the slave trade for the slow progress in the scientific development of African medical system. In most cases, scientific development is brought about by the daring and adventurous youthful mind. During the period of slave trade which spanned late 15th and early 19th Centuries, able-bodied young men and women were illicitly carried from Africa especially the western and eastern coasts to the West Indies. Consequently, African societies were left with predominantly old and too young minds. Moreover, the insecurity and instability which characterized the period did not augur well even for inquisitive people to direct their minds towards scientific development and growth. So devastating is the effect of colonialism and slavery that an American journalist writing on the effect of colonialism on the Africans remarks:

> The colonialists left behind some schools and roads, some post offices and bureaucrats. But their cruelest legacy on the African continent was a lingering inferiority complex, a confused sense of identity. After all, when people are told for a century that they're not as clever or capable as their masters, they eventually start to believe it.[23]

Ngugi Wa Thiong'o examines the slavery and colonialism in Africa and likens their cumulative effects to a cultural bomb; the effect of which is to annihilate the African belief in their names, languages, heritage, capacities, unity and, fundamentally, in themselves.[24] Walter Rodney, on the other hand, attributes the notion of superiority claim of the colonialists over the Africans to the effect of the slave trade. He argues that no people can enslave another for centuries without emerging with superiority and pride.[25]

However, Ivan Van Sertima, writing on the state of emergency all over Africa consequent on the trans-Atlantic slave trade and colonialism, asserts that:

No human disaster... can equal in dimension of destructiveness, the cataclysm that shook Africa. We are all familiar with the slave trade and the traumatic effect of this on the transplanted black, but few of us realize what horrors were wrought on Africa itself. Vast populations were uprooted and displaced, whole generations disappeared, European diseases descended like the plagues, decimating both cattle and people. Cities and towns were abandoned, family networks disintegrated, kingdoms crumbled, the thread of cultural and historical continuity were so savagely torn asunder that henceforth, one would have to think of two Africas: the one before and the one after the Holocaust. [26]

The slave trade was sustained by the theory of providential design. The theory argues that the enslavement of Africans and the subsequent colonization of the continent were due to God's providence. That God had designed the slave trade as a means of raising new African-Americans into Christianity. The slave trade had come to an end after the settlement and christianization of Africans in America so that the civilized and Christianized Americans and Africans could "bring it (the continent) to Christ". This theological justification of slavery and colonialism was acceptable to many people. [27] In addition to the providential design theory was the philosophical justification for slavery. Thus Hegel rationalized and legitimatized every European myth about Africa. For instance, he argued that Egypt, the cradle of civilization was not part of Africa; that North Africa was in Europe; that Africa was the home of ravenous beasts and snakes of all types; that the African is not a human being. Therefore, it was only slavery that could elevate him to the status of a lower human being. From this premise, Hegel concluded that slavery was good for the Africans. [28]

The Europeans were not alone in the justification of slave trade. Walter Rodney gave an example of a West African who wrote his doctoral thesis in Latin legitimizing slavery. In his thesis, he argued that slavery was justified because it brought the primitive African out of the dark jungle into the light of modern civilization. [29] The period of the slave trade in Africa compared to some extent with the dark ages (500-800 AD) [30] in Medieval Europe when the Goths, Franks, Vandals and Saxons (all barbarians) who were masters of Europe, could not read and write. They were, therefore, unaware of the civilizations of Greece and Rome. [31]

DEFINITIONS

Traditions

The *Concise Oxford Dictionary* defines tradition as "opinion or belief or custom handed down from ancestors to posterity especially orally or by practice" while the *Dictionary of Social Sciences* edited by Julius Could *et. al.* defines tradition as "the transmission, usually orally, whereby modes of activity or taste or belief are handed down (given across) from one generation to the next and thus perpetuated". When applied to social institutions, tradition is the vehicle through which every child learns something of the mores and stock of the accumulated knowledge and prejudices of his forefathers.

Funk and Wagnalls *International Standard Dictionary*, on the other hand, defines traditions as the transmission of knowledge, opinions, doctrines, customs, practices etc., from generation to generation, originally by word of mouth and by example; that which is so transmitted; body of beliefs and usage handed down from generation to generation; also any particular story, belief or usage so handed down; hence remembrance or recollection existing as by transmission.

Traditional medicinewhich is the cognate of tradition denotes the transmission of the values, activities, mores or beliefs from one generation to another. Essentially, tradition denotes the transmission of values, activities and beliefs from one generation to another orally or through practice. Tradition, therefore, does not involve the transmission of knowledge and so on through documentation.

Medicine

The *Concise Oxford Dictionary* defines medicine as "an art of restoring and preserving health especially by means of remedial substance and regulation of diet opposed to surgery and obstetrics. From the perspective of the less-developed societies, it defines medicines in terms of spells, charms, fetish. This is an attempt to relegate the medical system of the less-developed societies into the background. This attitude was occasioned by the superiority complex of the Euro-American scholars which was a bane to their understanding of the culture and religion of the people. Urhobo medicine is more than spells and charms .

According to the *Webster's New Twentieth Century Dictionary*, medicine is the "science and art of diagnosing, treating, curing and preventing disease, relieving pain, and improving and preserving health". It is the branch of the science which uses drugs, diets and so on as distinguished especially from surgery and obstetrics. It is also defined as "any drug or other substance used in treating disease, healing or relieving pain. It goes further to define medicine among North American Indians as any object, spell, rite and so on that is supposed to have natural or supernatural powers as a remedy, preventive and so on".

Chambers Twentieth Century Dictionary defines medicine as "any substance used (especially) internally for the treatment or prevention and cure of disease especially a non-surgical; a charm, magic, anything of magic power".

This definition has not brought out clearly the difference between medicine and magic. There are magical medicines which are used for the treatment, prevention or cure of diseases. Magical medicines involve the communication of incantations in them and it is difficult to say whether the efficacy of the medicine is in the active ingredients of the *materia medica* or in the incantations. Maclean designates such medicine as irrational.

Parrinder [32] in an attempt to clearly define medicine in the African context sees it as covering both natural healing agencies such as leaves, roots and so on and the invocation of magical or spiritual influences that are thought to be associated with them. Parrinder's emphasis is on healing.

Metuh, on the other hand, defines medicine in the African belief system as anything that can be used to heal, kill, secure power, health, fertility, personality or moral reforms. To him, medicine includes drugs for curing and preventing disease as well as objects with magical effects. [33] Thus making medicine among the Igbo has wider connotation than that suggested by the English translation. Metuh further observes that *Igwo Ogwu* (making medicine) includes herbal as well as psychotherapeutical and spiritual techniques, Medicine (*Ogwu*) does not only include herbal mixtures but also magical objects, incantations and rites capable of changing the human condition for the better or worse. [34]

Metuh's definition has not distinguished between medicine and sorcery. Medicine is generally accepted as means of preserving life. Hence the practitioners of medicine are proud of their profession. On the other hand, sorcerers are usually feared in every community and their activities are performed in secret and at night. The Urhobo call medicine and magical medicine *umu*, *umwu*, *or uhuvwu* depending on dialectical differentiation while witchcraft and sorcery are called *Orha.*

Perhaps it is in an attempt to portray this difference that Dopamu defines medicine as "the art of using the available resources of nature to prevent, treat or cure disease. It is an art aimed at restoring and preserving health by means of medicament. Medicine, therefore, is both therapeutic and prophylactic" (curative and preventive) [35].

To Idowu, medicine involves the restoration and preservation of health. Hence he says "it is logical that the preservation of health is mentioned after the mentioning of restoration because man must have learnt that health could be lost or impaired only through practical experience." To him, the purpose of medicine is "essentially to help the body to help itself." It is curative in that it helps the body return to its normal state. It is also preventive in that it builds up resistance against infection". [36]

On the whole, it is Dopamu's definition of medicine that relates to the Urhobo concept of medicine. Medicine in the Urhobo context can be defined as the art of using available resources of nature to prevent, and cure disease, enhance life and means of achieving one's aspiration. Thus medicine includes all magical preparations that prevent, cure, enhance life and assist in achieving one's aspiration.

Traditional Medicine

Mume[37] defines traditional medicine as the transmission by word of mouth and by example the knowledge and practice based on customary methods of natural healing or treatment of disease while Sofowora defines traditional medicine as "the total combination of knowledge and practice, whether explicable or not, used in diagnosing, preventing or eliminating a physical, mental or social disease, and which may rely exclusively on past experience and observation handed down from generation to generation, verbally or in writing. [38]

Among the various definitions of medicine and traditional medicine, Dopamu's definition of medicine and Sofowora's definition of traditional medicine are appropriate to the Urhobo concept of traditional medicine. Urhobo traditional medicine is the medical system practised by our progenitors and transmitted from one generation to another. Some of the procedures in the preparation and administration of magical medicine are inexplicable.

Magic

Awolalu and Dopamu define magic as an attempt by man to tap and control the supernatural powers or resources of the universe for his own benefits.[39] Magic operates on the basis that there are supernatural powers in the universe which can be harnessed and manipulated for man's end. Thus magic refers to "the art of using available resources of nature to procure non-therapeutic needs of man, either for good or for bad. It is the art of influencing the course of events by means of supernatural communications and manifestation of power, or by means of occult control of nature and invocation of particular aids". [40]

From the definition, there are good magic or magical medicine and bad magic or sorcery. Good magic caters for the well-being of the individual and community. In this context, the Urhobo call it *umu/umwu/uhuvwu*. Thus, the Urhobo have magical preparations against witchcraft, *inewhere, enivwovo* (magical preparation for love), *ekpofia* (magical preparation against untoward occurrences, bullets and cutlass), *useki* (magical preparation for successful business including hunting and trading), *umu rariebe* (magical preparation for retentive memory prepared for students), *umu edjo* (magical preparation for winning court cases).

Among the Urhobo, the distinction drawn between medicine and magical medicine is strange if we accept the definition of medicine as "the art of using the available resources of nature to prevent, treat or cure diseases. It is the art of restoring and preserving health by means of medicament". [41] For instance, there is a medicine for migraine. The *materia medica* may possess the active principles for relieving the pain but it must be applied when the sun is setting between 4.00 and 5.00 p.m. It must be performed outside with the patient facing the sun. The remedy is rubbed on the seat of the pain. The patient is then asked to indicate where he feels the pain again. This is repeated until he is finally asked to shake the head and indicate the seat of the pain. This is done until the patient declares that he does not feel the pains again. [42] Una Maclean designates such treatment as magico-rational. It is magical because of the position of the patient and the time when the remedy is administered; it is rational because the medicine contains the active agents.

In the aetiology in traditional medicine, ailments that are caused supernaturally and socially/preternaturally require a combination of rational and preternatural treatment often referred to as magical treatment. Una Maclean [43] describes magical treatment as examples of irrationality and malpractice, a mixture of superstition, deliberate deception and ignorance while E. B. Tylor[44] describes it as "a monstrous farrago containing no truth or value whatsoever".

However, Shorter has warned against this sceptical attitude found among the foreigners and the social scientists that though by training and profession they should be sceptical, they should also preserve an open mind; that they should be ready to encounter irrefutable evidence that magic really works; and that events anticipated in symbolic rite really occur.[45]

Ayoade [46] identifies four major principles upon which preternatural African medicine operates. These principles include, the principle of similarity, contact, unusualness and transferability; and he goes on to explicate each principle. Magical or preternatural treatment is the point of departure between traditional and orthodox western medical systems.

So bewildered were the Christian missionaries about the Yoruba use of magical medicines or charms that they preached against it and sought to convert them into Christianity. But the Yoruba who have implicit belief in its curative, protective and destructive functions viewed the missionaries' attempt as reducing their converts to women. As they express it: "what kind of man could stand firm in this evil world without the private fortification given him by some *oogun* or the other, tied to his waist, worn in a ring, swallowed at dawn or recited in a spell".[47]

Oduyoye bemoans the adverse effect of Christianity and education on Yoruba medicine, especially the good magical medicine. However, she encourages the consultation of medicine men whose medical skill she considers as a share of God's spirit but condemns belief in magicians and sorcerers who wreak vengeance or punish the innocent with their power. She asserts that:

> Of all the aspects of African traditional beliefs that we must encourage our people to jettison, belief in magic is one in which we can have no hesitation. We will still need to consult medicine men and medical specialists. [48]

But Oguakwa [49] and Olusegun Obasanjo[50] posit that humanity will rejoice if magical knowledge, that is, the destructive aspect can be employed to liberate man from the clutches of apartheid; that any time this happens, Africa shall have launched "The African Renaissance in Medicine". Oguakwa is, however, worried about the absence of acceptable explanation (scientific or otherwise) for the demonstrable feats. Dr Nnamdi Azikiwe has once echoed the same point that:

> Unless the African scientist could invent a fourth form or nature of matter which is unknown in the realm of pure science, whatever conclusions he had built upon the basis of his theories of medicine must fall flat. This does not mean that it is not true. It is simply this; that this brand of African medicine is demonstrable.[51]

Oguakwa, Obasanjo and Azikiwe are contemplative of the possibility of transferring the bad magical aspect of traditional medicine to a larger scale and introducing science and technology into it so that Africa could become one of the world powers. To achieve this objective, Oguakwa suggests that Africans should imitate the Chinese who studied the scientific aspects of their heritage and finally developed acupuncture which is today a living science.[52] He is very optimistic that if the documented and undocumented works of our progenitors in the area of traditional medicine can be intensively and continuously investigated by Africans, a discovery of similar potential as acupuncture could also be made by Africans.[53]

Shorter, arguing from anthropological perspective, categorizes magic or medicine into good and bad. That while good magic or medicine brings about good effects — cure, protection, profit to a person or community; bad magic or medicine produces bad effect — harm, destruction or hindrance.[54] Magical medicine is usually accompanied with the words of intention or incantations.

Sorcery

The *Concise Oxford Dictionary* defines a sorcerer as a user of magic arts while the *Advanced Learner's Dictionary* defines it as a man who practises with the help of evil spirits. The definition of the *Concise Oxford Dictionary* does not indicate whether magic is good or bad but the definition presupposes that magic art means evil art.

Parrinder differentiates a sorcerer from a witch. To him, a witch is incapable of doing what he or she is supposed to do and has no real existence while a sorcerer uses magic to kill his neighbour.[55] Parrinder's view that a witch has no real existence is strange to the Africans. Witches have existence and their confessional statements testify to their existence.

Awolalu and Dopamu define sorcery as an employment of bad or illicit magic especially meant to kill, harm, destroy life and property, to make a happy destiny an unhappy one, to disrupt the well-being of the individual and society. Thus, a sorcerer is a person who uses bad magic. Characteristically, a sorcerer is evil, feared and often hated because of his anti-social activities which are usually performed in darkness.[56] Invocations and incantations are mostly employed by sorcerers.

Dopamu views sorcery as a means or weapon which the poor use against the rich, weak against strong, the unfavoured against favoured, the commoner against the noble and the envious against the lucky ones. To Dopamu, sorcery like witchcraft has social function and that it is a means of providing something to blame when things go awry and a means of explaining social tensions.

Dopamu attributes the use of sorcery to lack of good neighbourliness which is inimical to societal peace.[57] Dopamu like Oduyoye feels that sorcery should be jettisoned so that atmosphere of friendliness where all will live and work in peace, love and harmony will prevail since power corrupts and absolute power corrupts absolutely.

EARLY VIEWS OF TRADITIONAL MEDICINE AND ITS PRACTITIONERS

The early anthropologists, ethnographers, traders and missionaries who undertook the study of traditional medicine and its practitioners looked at the African world with different cultural lenses and could not understand the African religion and philosophical framework in which the Africans perceived existence. According to Achebe, "each mode is a lens through which man, in a given culture, views his world. Each cultural lens enables it to see only a certain part of the world. If one wore different lens, one would see a different world"[58] The traditional medicine and its practitioners were thus dubbed superstitious, fetish, animistic, witch-doctor and magician. Kalu opines that medicine men were dubbed witch-doctors because it was the element of magic in African medicine which captured more of the foreigners' attention.[59] The popular image of the traditional medicine and its practitioners is well-articulated by Iwu thus:

> The popular image of the African medicine men as that of a fabled witch-doctor with his exotic paraphernalias of feathers, cowries and animal skin muttering meaningless incantations and dispensing worthless potions to equally ignorant clients. Even the herbs they dispense are considered harmful and when they are found efficacious, the detractors of traditional medicine are quick to dismiss them as chance discovery. The incantations and the rhythm of drums are said to be weird sounds and part of the mumbo-jumbo designed to hoodwink the superstitious savages who are under their spell.[60]

In consonance with the above view, Gelfand designates medicine man witch-doctors and uses the two terms interchangeably.[61] Thus in his book, *The African Witch*[62] he specifically uses witch-doctor for medicine man. Galfand accuses medicine man of merely treating symptoms because of their inability to link together symptom and sign. Gelfand has erred in his assessment of the medicine man. The medicine man does only deal with symptoms but approaches his treatment through the multi-dimensional factors that cause diseases.[62] Thus medicine men are described as physicians, psychotherapists and spirit healers. As Mbiti aptly observes "on the whole, the medicine man gives much time and personal attention to the patient which enables him to penetrate deep into the psychological state of the patient."[63] In the same vein, Oguakwa asserts that an Africanist is fully aware that disease hardly comes singly, that if a sick person complains of anaemia, the Africanist, from experience treats malaria and worm invasion if his treatment is to be efficacious.[64]

This meticulous attention is not only given to symptoms but to all the aspects of the disease. Bibeau, G. *et.al.* writing on the Zaire medicine men posits that in diagnosing an illness, healers often take into account two basic signs: body temperature and the quantity of blood. Healers attach great importance to physical symptom and focus their attention on changes in the various parts of the body affected by the illness.[65] Ademuwagun who has carefully and critically studied the diagnostic methodological system of the medicine man also observes:

> A critical analysis of the diagnostic methods show that the traditional health personnel are astute and shrewd behavioural scientists of no mean capacity. As pragmatists in their profession, their brand of behavioural science is in consonance with specific skill and well–calculated socio-cultural and psychological situational reality in patient's total environment.[66]

This misconception and the subsequent derogatory terms used in describing traditional medicine and its practitioner made the missionaries view them as targets of attack and campaigns of vilification. They were, therefore, regarded as the main propagators of superstition and magic and were inelegantly dubbed with all sorts of designations: magicians, sorcerers, witch-doctors and witch-hunters.[67] But today missionaries and others have been proved wrong in their employment of these perjorative terms; hence Evans-Pritchard's warning is noteworthy. He has observed how unreliable the statements of the early explorers, traders, and others on religious matters of the so-called primitive people they had visited are. He, therefore, warns that statements about people's religious beliefs must always be treated with the greatest caution. These religious beliefs, he posits, cannot be observed directly and that their understanding requires a thorough knowledge of a people's language and also an awareness of the entire system of ideas of which any particular belief is a part. He suggests that the removal of a concept, image or word from the set of beliefs and practices to which it belongs renders it meaningless.[68]

Inflamed by the bloated ideas of the superiority of western civilization and science especially medical science, the early traders, missionaries, ethnographers and anthropologists did not bother to pry into the traditional medical system to see whether the medicines were efficacious. For most part, traditional medicines were depicted in their writings as inefficacious. Ezeabasili writing from a nationalistic perspective has this point against them and he dismissed their theses as propaganda. [69] But today, the indispensability of a people's worldview in the effective management of disease as practised by the African medical experts from time immemorial has long been realized by western medical experts and Africans trained in the western medical system—Lambo, Una Maclean and educational psychologist, Christie Achebe. As Lambo puts it:

> Man's belief concerning his culture...environment determines to a large extent the interpretation of concept of health and diseases and the methods of therapy to be employed in resolving life crisis... Medicine in a broad sense can be regarded as a constituent part of social institutions since it is bound up with the whole interpretation of life.

O.U Kalu writing on the significance of the African worldview in understanding its medical system asserts:

> African medicine can only be properly understood in its complete cultural context since the way in which people respond to illness or misfortune in any culture is inevitably related to the whole religious and philosophical framework in which they perceive existence. [70]

Christie Achebe also writing on the Igbo concept of Ogbanje in her book *The World of Ogbanje* [71] has discussed extensively the signal position of worldview in the comprehension of a people's mode of perception and conceptualization of phenomena and existence. Christie Achebe, like other scholars, views the misconception and the pejorative terms used in describing traditional medicine and its practitioners as emanating from the fact that the early anthropologists, ethnographers, traders and others wore different lenses with which they viewed the traditional religion and culture.

Today the medicine men have taken their proper place among the professionals and the traditional medicine has been proved (beyond any reasonable doubt) to be efficacious. Thus Harrison in his article "Traditional Healer as a Source of Traditional and Contemporary Powers", carefully describes them as belonging to the class of professionals. He defines the "class" as a number of persons sharing a common style of life due to economic pursuits based on the monopoly of property, goods and services, and that birth, disease, disorder and death are universals in human experience. The healer, he contends, is a member of a universal class in that societies have individuals who treat disruptive experience. [72]

PRACTITIONERS OF TRADITIONAL MEDICINE

The praxis of traditional medicine is within the domain of three specialists — the medicine man, diviner and priest which include both men and women. Mbiti (1973:167) and Kokwaro (1976:4) observe that women often specialise in obstetrics, gynaecology, paediatrics, circumcision of girls and other general treatment while their male counterparts handle special cases like leprosy, abscess, gonorrhoea and so on. Awolalu and Dopamu (1979), Oliver (1960) [73], Una Maclean(1971), Dopamu (n.d) and Bibeau *et al.* also lend their support to the involvement of women in the traditional medical system but Maclean, who carried out a similar study in Ghana as she did in Ibadan, observes that women are more involved in Ghana than in Nigeria. Dopamu also observes that women tend to restrict themselves to therapeutics, especially for the ailments of women and children. [74]

Each of these specialists has his distinctive role to perform in the traditional medical system. The African perception of the aetiology in traditional medicine underscores the role of each specialist. The medicine man basically heals through the utilization of medicine; the diviner through divination while the priest handles diseases emanating from guilt against the gods, ancestors and humanity which involve offering of sacrifice. As Metuh rightly observes:

> The Igbo distinguish between the *dibia afa*, diviner and *dibia ogwu* medicine man. Both are *dibia* (healer). However, whereas the one heals by *afa*, divination, the other heals by *ogwu*, medicine. The diviner sees the spiritual and material factors involved in a given situation. The medicine man applies the remedies if they are within the scope of his medical practice. In other words, the diviner is a diagnostician-psychotherapist-spirit healer. [75]

Ezeanya examines the ministration of the priest in the traditional medical system. He opines that the priest is mainly responsible for the performance of sacrifice arising from abominable offences committed against the supersensible and man. He vouches that:

> A person who has committed an abominable act detestable to the divinities and men is really a sick person. Such acts like stealing, particularly of commodities like yams, fowls and goats, murder, incest, adultery committed by a wife and such-like offences are abominable acts and call for the healing from ministry of the priest. [76]

Opoku also concedes that both priest and herbalist are involved in the traditional medical system.

Medicine making in the African context comprehends more than the western usage. Hence, Metuh asserts that medicine making embraces herbal medicine as well as psychotherapeutical and spiritual healing techniques. That *ogwu* (medicine) includes herbal mixtures, magical objects, incantations and rites which are capable of changing the human condition for the better or the worse. [77]

Functionally, the medicine man deals with both the natural and supernatural diseases while the diviner is mainly involved in supernatural diseases. Supernatural diseases are characterized by their extreme infractoriness to proven efficacious treatment, severeness, chronic or exotic. In such cases, recourse is had on divination to pry into the causes of the disease. The history of the disease is usually fed on the divination board. As Ilogu asserts: "Divination in the case of illness nearly always, leads to finding out what spirit had been wronged and what human relationship had been strained. Sacrifice and propitiation accompanied whatever herbal medicine is given to ensure proper cure". [78]

Talbot focuses on the use of divination as chiefly to discover causes of sickness and the appropriate method of cure of the former case, to find out the wishes of the gods and ancestors and to unveil the future.[79] Campbell in the same way writing on divination among the Ngwakatse observes that a large proportion of the population employ the services of a diviner at all moments of crisis or decision especially in seeking solution to the cause of inexplicable occurences or sickness, or to determine the right steps to be taken to bring a doubtful issue to a successful conclusion. [80] Campbell's statement indicates the vital position of the diviner in African societies. Hence, Mbiti (1969:166) describes the diviner and the medicine man as the greatest friends of the African communities.

Diviners are often accused of having a chain of informants and a good eye on the on-goings of the communities as means of obtaining information. On the other hand, it is also argued that the diviner throws some leading questions to the enquirer which enable him to appropriately assess the situation. It is for this reason, the diviner is imbued with a good knowledge of psychology. Parrinder (1969:137) aptly describes the diviner:

> It is certain that they sometimes seem to gain knowledge of people's deeds or the whereabout of their lost or stolen goods, by methods which are not easily explicable. Some would say that they have secret agents to listen to village gossips and watch suspected people; others claim that they practise telepathy and have powers of prevision.[81]

While we accept Parrinder's statement, nobody doubts the presence of charlatans in the divination profession but it is not always that this happens. Hence, S.U. Erivwo writing on *Epha* (divination) among the Urhobo observes that while this may happen, it is not always the case because "diviners have also been known to tell their clients the object of their mission at their appearance, even before they have had time to say anything; a phenomenon which would indicate that there is some element of telepathy in the process of divination."[82]

Summarising the functions of diviners in African societies, Mbiti sees them as performing the roles of judges, counsellors, suppliers of assurance and confidence during people's crisis, pastors, advisers, seers and solvers of problem.[83]

Call to the Profession

Traditional medical practitioners — medicine men, diviners and priests — receive their call to the profession through tutelary divinity of medicine and divination. The tutelary divinity of medicine and divination among the Igbo is *Agwu* while among the Yoruba, *Osanyin* and *Orunmila* are the divinities for medicine and divination respectively. The call comes through indication in dreams, apparitions, divination, mysterious events or a concatenation of two or more of these. Arinze (1970:64), Isichei (1978:172), Metuh (1981:68: 1985: 153-65) and Ezeanya (1978:4) among others give credence to the above assertion. Isichei, for instance, describes how *Araba* a divinity among the Ika people of Delta State of Nigeria, chooses her chief priest. It is believed that the chosen one is often known through certain violent changes which occur in the individual. The chief priest she studied received his call through series of dreams. [84]

Arinze is specific about the call of a diviner by asserting that a *dibia*-to-be is usually possessed by spirit of the *Agwu*, the special spirit of *ndi dibia*, the spirit of giddiness, rascality, discomposure, confusion and forgetfulness. Usually one or more of these characteristics are noticed in a neophyte,[85] while Metuh remarks that the *dibia ogwu* medicine man like the diviner is summoned to his profession by *Agwu*, the patron divinity of diviners and medicine men.[86] Westerman writing on the three medical specialists opines: "It is natural that when a person has been summoned by a deity so directly, he should feel personally and forever bound to it, and that such an experience may be a turning-point in his life."[87]

Secondly, the profession may be inherited from a father, grandfather or mother. Metuh (1985:60) says that among the Igbo, the profession is inherited through one's matriclan and that if one is possessed by *Agwu*, it eventually means that there has been a history of divination practice in one's matriclan. It is only those who minister to *Agwu* that are possessed by *Agwu*. Among the Yoruba, heredity is considered enough condition for becoming a medicine man. Maclean[88] and Prince[89] indicate that among the Yoruba, medicine men come, in most cases, from families with long medical traditions. These families are noteworthy in that they are contemporary products of extensive medical lore. Mume pursuing the argument further states that he became a naturopathist because his grand maternal cousin was a medicine man of repute from whom he acquired the art.[90] He was always given the opportunity to sit close to his master throughout the period of training and was thus able to learn the names of more than nine hundred different plants and their medicinal usage.

Thirdly, there are cases of persons carried into the spirit world and were taught the art of medicine there. Ayoade reports of Mr. Aladokun of Ikirun who was carried to the spirit world where he was taught the secrets of the profession.

Ayoade contends that such spirit-disciples are endowed with powers to cause things to happen or to prevent them from happening. Such powers, he opines, are personal and not transmissible for the power is in their touch which gives the desired effect. [91] Idowu[92] is of the same opinion.

Finally, one may become a medicine man out of one's volition and interest by apprenticing himself to a well-known medicine man. Among the Bambara, Campbell asserts, the art of divination is not hereditary although sons may learn it from their fathers; but that in normal cases a man apprentices himself to a successful diviner who spends two to three years in teaching him the art. [93]

Training

Scholars of Afrel and Culture, whether foreign or indigenous, unanimously assent that African medical practitioners undergo a period of tutelage under a successful and experienced medical practitioner. The period of training varies from an aggregate of people to another. Nadel (1954: 17-21; 133-162)[94]; Green (1964: 54)[95]; Mbiti (1969: 166-72)[96]; (1975: 150-5)[97]; Evans-Pritchard (1976: 177-204)[98] Opoku (1978: 148-151)[99] among others, lend their support to the fact that African medical practitioners undergo a period of apprenticeship.

Evans-Pritchard specifically asserts that the recruitment and training of medicine men among the Azande is expensive and tedious. Prince who studied the Yoruba traditional medical system contends that the period of training varies from three to twenty years while Maclean's (1969: 76) opinion corroborates Prince's point of view.

From the review of some of the related literature, it is evident that the African medical system and its practitioner are unique and, of right as a profession just as the practice of orthodox medicine is a profession. The initial pejorative terms used in describing traditional medicine and its practitioner were due mainly to error of judgement arising from the fact that foreigners wore different cultural lenses with which they viewed the African world and its phenomena.

CHAPTER TWO

Definition and Taxonomy

INTRODUCTION

Traditional and orthodox medical systems are two different and distinct medical systems practised in two different cosmologies. Thus, the Urhobo medical system is based on the Urhobo cosmology while the practice of orthodox medical system is based on the western cosmology. However, because they both are of the same medical profession, they have the same register. Some of the medical terms have been defined in the context of orthodox medicine. Since Urhobo traditional medicine is quite distinct from the orthodox medical system, such medical terminologies will be defined in relation to Urhobo perspective.

This chapter examines the Urhobo cosmology which is the explanation of the universe around it. The adoption of comparative analysis warrants the examination of Urhobo cosmology vis-a-vis western scientific cosmology as these affect their medical systems. This will enhance the indication of points of continuity and discontinuity. In the praxis of Urhobo medical systems, the nosology is carried out according to their aetiology. In the same vein, the treatment modality of an ailment is a function of the nature of the illness. Thus, the aetiology and nosology of disease are also investigated. Attempt will also be made to probe into the various Urhobo therapeutic methods since the nature of the ailment determines the type of therapeutic method to be employed. Finally, the taxonomy of Urhobo medicine is discussed.

The apprehension of a people warrants the study of their cosmology since this underscores their thought forms, norm of behaviour and their philosophical frame of mind. The British colonial officers realized the signal role of cosmology in the understanding of a people; hence they undertook the study of the Igbo cosmology with a view to understanding them better so that effective and efficient colonial administration might be carried out. This concept is well-illustrated by the Intelligence Report on the Igbo quoted by A. Afigbo: The fact was that the very difficulty they experienced in governing the Igbo forced the colonial officers to conduct some research in Igbo institutions and worldview in the hope of finding the key to the situation.[1]

20

Ejizu opines that such various researches undertaken by the colonial officers and schools were informed by their desire to find indigenous socio-political leadership which would serve as a prop for hoisting their policy of Indirect System of Colonial Administration of Igboland.[2]

Understanding Medicine: Worldview Approach

Worldview is used interchangeably with cosmology. Cosmology, according to Webster's Third *New International Dictionary* (Vol. 1,p. 154) is "a branch of systematic philosophy that deals with the character of the universe as a *cosmos* by combining speculative metaphysics and scientific knowledge, especially a branch of philosophy that deals with the processes of nature and the relation of its parts".

The *Oxford English Dictionary* (Vol. 3) defines cosmology as "derived from the Greek word, *Cosmologia. Cosmos* means "word" and *logia* denotes "discourse". It is the science or theory of the universe as an ordered whole, and the general laws which govern it. It is also a particular account or system of the universe and its laws". Thus, worldview deals with how man perceives the world in relation to himself. Metuh defines worldview as: "The complex of a people's belief about the origin, structure and organization of the universe, and the laws governing the interaction of beings in it".[3]

O.U. Kalu defines and discusses the function of worldview as: "The intellectual or rational explanations of the order which undergird human lives and environments. This undergirding order is derivable from myths, taboos, customs and proverbs of a community"[4].

The functions of a worldview include: assistance of man in the explanation of reality, thereby making him feel secure in a world of uncertainty; helping man to predict space-time events and also enabling man to exercise control over these events. To these may be added the fourth function; that is, one's world-view which encapsulates one's attitude, opinions, values and concepts which influence one's mode of thinking, taking decisions, behaving and defining events, thereby affording man a means of conceptualizing or thinking about other people and their world. However, Achebe argues that this conceptualization of other people and their world might be performed erroneously since different cultures have different ways of ordering their world. Each mode is a lens through which man in a given culture, views his world. Each cultural lens enables man to see only a certain part of the world. Thus if one wore a different lens, one would see a different world.[5]

Animalu sees worldview as a means of explaining the how-and-why of daily existence and therefore, the major cultural ingredient of every society. He contends that these worldviews emanate from experiences full of dramatic events giving rise to customs or totems of one kind or the other; these symbols or totems in turn give rise to thoughts which in turn give rise to customs and codes of the society. The success of a worldview depends on its degree of internalization from childhood process of socialization to the extent that it is not questioned. Its manifestations are the various forms of artistic expressions.[6]

The understanding of a people's cosmology is, therefore, vital in comprehending the people themselves. Worldview elucidates such questions as why people behave in a particular way, think differently from others and their philosophy of life is distinct from others. It is an attempt to explicate these points that Uchendu remarks: "To know how people view the world around them is to understand how they evaluate life and people's evaluation of life (both temporal and non-temporal) provides them with a "Charter" of action, a guide to behaviour."[7]

URHOBO COSMOLOGY

Oghene: The Supreme Being

The Urhobo believe in a Supreme Being who created the world and everything in it. They call Him *Oghene, Uku, Agbadagbruru, Osonobruwhe, Obe Ode Otakponarhurhu* but *Oghene* is the commonly used name. Each people has a local name for the Supreme Being. The Igbo call Him *Chukwu* while the Yoruba call Him *Olodumare*. As Ezea remarks: "Every nation under heaven has the consciousness of one great Maker of things. This consciousness we talk of as the revelation content given to human beings, by the Creator, the Creator left His creation full of wonders".[8]

Bradbury says that the Urhobo worship a high god, *Oghene,* who is the creator of the world and of life and death.[9] The idea of a high god was coined by the westerners to differentiate God as conceived by the Africans from their God of the Holy Bible. This high god, the westerners argued, was peculiar to the Africans and by implication each people in Africa had a high god.

This distinction makes it evident that there are Supreme Beings for the Christians, Muslims, the secularized westerners and the Africans. This statement clearly betrays the ignorance and the superiority complex of the westerners for Afrel. It has, however, been discovered that there are no high gods in Africa. It is the only one God of the universe who makes Himself manifest to the different peoples and races of the world. All races and people are capable of experiencing God's self-revelation but the difference is that the response to this self-disclosure varies from locality to locality in accordance with the intellectual and spiritual abilities of the people.[10] A. O. Erhueh has argued that God reveals Himself to all people in the worthy elements of their cultures not only in the very nature of those persons (since all were created image *Dei*) but in all their activities which enable them to develop humane qualities and the humanization of the world.[11] St.

Augustine also expressed the same point in his statement that: "God speaks to his people in the way the people speak to themselves". [12]

Uku, Agbadagbruru and Osonobruwhe, Obe Odeotakporhurhu indicate the omnipresence, almightiness, power, majesty and benevolence of God. The omnipresence is clearly demonstrated by associating the sky with God and is even called *Oghene.* This attribute of *Oghene* is well-brought out when the people say: *"Ode Otakporhurhu* (the plantain leaf that is big enough to shelter the whole world)". [13]

The royalty, majesty and almightiness of *Oghene* is referred to when the Urhobo address *Oghene* as *Uku* which is the cognate of *Uku Okpolokpolo* the way the Bini address their *Oba.* [14] and *Obe Ode Otakporhurhu* (the plantain leaf sufficiently big to shelter the whole world) or *Ohwovo or tota otu nyo* (the only man who speaks and the multitude hear). These attributes closely associate thunder and lightning with *Oghene's* speech. The attributes of love and justice are also ascribed to *Oghene.* Thus, the Urhobo say *Amwa Oghene bru k' ohwo oye te ohwo vwo rhue and orhie r'Oghene bruru amrasa muo ra-a* (It is the cloth that God cuts for one which is all sufficient to clothe one) and (in God's judgement there is no appeal) whenever they feel that enough love and justice have not been adequately demonstrated.

The attributes of *Oghene* are evident in the theophorous names which the Urhobo give their children-*Oghenekohwo* (God is the giver), *Oghaneochuko* (God is the helper) *Oghenemine* (It is God I look up to), *Oghenevwohwodua* (It is only God that makes one great), *Oghenebrume* (God has vindicated me) and such other names.

As the Creator of all things, the Urhobo call *Oghene Orovwakpo, vwerivwi ve odjuvwu* (the owner of *akpo* (world) *erivwi* (the spirit world) and *odjuvwu* (the spirit world) is in most cases used to denote where *Oghene* is). As the creator of all things visible and invisible, the Urhobo refer to Him as *Omemamo* (Creator of all things) and as the creator of man, He is called *Omaromohwo*. As the Creator, the Urhobo conceive Him as a Moulder. Hence, in most cases when an unusual event (sudden death of a prosperous young man or a disaster) occurs, the Urhobo express their surprise by saying: *Emu ra mrere-e ye Oghene maro-o* [15] (Whatever is not seen was never created by God)".

Oghene as the Creator also created the *edjo* and *erha* (divinities), *irhi* (plural of *erhi*-spirits), and *ohwo* (man), *eravwe* (animals), *irhe* (trees), *irhie* (rivers) and other beings or phenomena in the universe. Thus, there are the physical *(akpo)* and the psychic *(erivwi)*, the visible *(oboramre)* and invisible *(obaramre-e)* and the social and the spiritual realms of existence.

The Urhobo do not, however, see these worlds as distinct from each other but are complementary. Talbot understood this complementarity of these worlds among the people of West Africa where the ancestral worship is predominant when he remarked that the dividing line between the dead and living is tenuous and that in the thinking and feeling of the West Africans, "the dead are not dead but living, and in full command of their faculties". [16] Ezeanya writing about the same concept among the Igbo asserts: "The veil that is drawn between the seen and the unseen is to the Igbo, a very thin veil so transparent that it is thought it can hardly be said to exist". [17]

S.U. Erivwo using the same argument to account for ancestral worship among the Urhobo opines that the living dead are separated only by a thin veil which is transparent especially to the *oboepha* (diviner). He contends that the communication between the living-dead and the *oboepha* (diviner) is due to this transparency of the separating line. This possibility or certainty of communication with the living-dead and the living through which the living solicit their assistance is the *raison d'etre* for the ancestor worship in Urhoboland. [18] Erivwo's argument does not only account for ancestor worship but also for all forms of saint worship and belief that some saints are patrons of safe journey: St. Jude, Virgin Mary, St. Peter, and St. Paul in Catholic and Anglicanism.

Oghene is believed to be the giver of the people's moral code and the *edjo, erha;* and *esemo* and *iniemo* (ancestors) are messengers and functionaries in His theocratic government of the universe. They are the custodians of the moral code. Thus, they are believed to punish an offender and bless those who uphold the morals. *Oghene*, as the creator forms the focal point in the Urhobo cosmology. Nobody requires any instruction about it. In fact, Ifesieh's remarks corroborate this view point in his discussion of the concept of God among the Igbo when he says that every Igbo imbibes the concept during his process of socialization and observation of the world around him. "In fact, this pivoted belief in *Chineke*, the Creator, is something one knows without being taught. One only needs to come to the age of reason and observe the world around one, the belief in the Supreme Being in Igbo religion as well as African religion is simply axiomatic because He is the focal point of Igbo theology". [19]

As the Creator and Omniscient God, *Oghene* sees the hearts of men and He is the Supreme Judge. Hence, the Urhobo give the name *Oghenebrorhie* (God is the Supreme and final judge) to their children when they feel cheated. He is the determiner and sustainer of the people's destiny and life. Thus, they believe that whatever they do, if it is to succeed, must be sanctioned by the Creator, the final judge and sustainer of their lives. However, *Oghene* is generally regarded as good.

Oghene is worshipped by the Urhobo against the casual observation of foreign observers. S. U. Erivwo asserts that the Urhobo do not only honour a Supreme Being but accord *Oghene* regular and frequent worship. Although, there are no temples and specialist priests to minister in His cult, there are altars erected for *Oghene*. Nabofa, [20] identifies three forms in which *Oghene* is at least worshipped but Erivwo identifies five forms of worship [21]

These are basically the perfunctory worship as indicated in spontaneous prayers when a man is saved from accident. The Urhoboman instantly acknowledges the almightiness and goodness of *Oghene* by saying *Oghene wo ru ru* (God has done well) while others who saw or heard about the incident would say *Akpevwoghene* (Thank God). Even in the face of the accident, the Urhoboman would say *Oghene biko sivwe* (God save me). These spontaneous prayers are indicative of the Urhoboman's recognition of the omnipotence, omnipresence and omniscience of *Oghene*.

Secondly, there is the regular worship of *Oghene* by the head of every family through the use of *orhe* (kaolin) every morning. The *orhe* is reduced to powder while it is on the palm and facing the east during sunrise, he prays to *Oghene* for the well-being of the members of his family and those of the extended family. He also prays to *Oghene* to punish his enemies including the witches by saying: *sivwi emo me sivwe ihwo eje. Ekevuovo me re ke oruimuemu-u* (save my children and everybody but 1 do not pray for the wicked). At the end of the prayer, he blows the powder towards the east. The *orhe* is a symbol of purity and using it in prayers evinces *Oghene*'s purity and the worshippers' belief that the *orhe* goes to *Oghene*.

The daily worship is always performed before the devoted worshipper speaks with any mortal. When the worshipper wakes up every morning, he takes a chewing stick and after he has brushed his teeth with it, looks to heaven with the chewing stick in his hand, and prays to *Oghene* beginning with *Oghene*'s praise names.

Oghene, ubi ukpabe

Obe ode oteakporhurhu.

The plantain leaf that is big enough

to shelter the whole world.

He then pours out his heart's desires and terminates the prayer by invoking the wrath of *Oghene* on his enemies.

Finally, the full and circumstantial worship of *Oghene* may be occasioned by a quarrel of wives in the compound (especially at night) or a member of the family may angrily invoke the wrath of *Oghene* and swear by him or *Osonobruhwe* as seen in a dream by any member of the family, especially the head. This worship is resemblance of the *esemo* (ancestor worship) in which a rich dish is prepared with either a goat or a rare fish normally *eba* or *erho* with live white chicken in attendance. The food is brought before the priest (usually the elderly man in the family) who is seated facing the altar where there is the *Orise* with all the family members sitting behind him. All the members would pray expressing their needs to *Oghene*. The elder rounds off by praying on behalf of the members present and absent as follows:

Osonobruhwe; Ovwatana Ovwaharena

We yere miakpo ve obo re hero eje
Avware ihwe eje koko rhe go we none
Wo da ta ne ado ka dua
Je erhuvwu na dia ki ihwo eje
Ohwo rota ne erhuvwu re`anere na je oye-e
Re oguonore ne oyovwi kihwo-eje-e
Wo re Osonobruwhe koye rie ohwo ye na
Wo ghare oghare ojewe vwo ke
Wo sio na ohri ravware
Asa rowo ma te, we mi sivwi te
Ihwo na eje ke tane, Ise.[22]

Osonobruhwe, Ovwatana Ovwaharena
You created the world and all its fullness
We are all assembled to worship you today
If you say one should be great, then one is great.
Let goodness be ours, not evil
Let this goodness extend to everyone
He who is not pleased with the goodness
Prayed for, it is you, *Osonobruwhe*, who knows such a person.
Give him the portion you consider apt for him.
Remove him from our midst.
Save all your creatures
(Lit: As many as you have created so may you save).
Everybody answers: Amen.

The food is then offered to *Oghene* while the white fowl whose legs are tied together is hung on the *Orise,* the symbol of *Oghene.* The remaining food is then communally eaten.

From the above analysis and observation, it is evident that what G. Parrinder said about the Ashanti is also applicable to the Urhobo, when he said that "The Ashanti are unique in West Africa not in honouring a Supreme Being, but in having temples, priests and altars for Him, and in fact, over the whole of tropical Africa, the only other people who seem to give similar attention to God are the *Kikuyu* of Kenya"[23].

Edjo and *Erha*: Divinities

The Urhobo believe that *Oghene* is not only the Creator and sustainer of the world but also the ultimate source and end of morality. He, therefore, created the *edjo* and *erha* (divinities) as His functionaries and intermediaries between Himself and man. Peculiar to the Urhobo is the fact that apart from *Oghene,* there is no divinity which the whole Urhobo worship together. This indicates that each of the twenty-two socio-political units has its own *edjo* and *erha* which aided them during their process of migration, settlement and wars of expansion. Myths abound which relate the roles such *edjo* and *erha* performed during such wars.

It is believed among the Urhobo that during the wars, *edjo* and *erha* rendered the guns, cutlasses and other weapons of the enemies ineffective; they made them panic-stricken before their devotees and revealed war tactics to them. For illustrative purpose, there is a myth among the Abraka people about how *Ovwuvwe*, their divinity, made *Avwaeke*, their progenitor flee from imminent death by sending the squirrel to warn him of an impending danger. This premonition made *Avwaeke* leave the area before the arrival of the Bini warriors.[24] In the same way, *Ifie* and *Igbodu* of *Arhavwarien* revealed to the *Ilotu* (warriors) that any time they were being pursued by enemies, they should hide in the bush, pluck some green leaves, put them in their mouth length-wise and invoke *Ifie* or *Igbodu* in their minds, and by that they would become invisible to their enemies. The appropriation of this power of camouflage is tailored to taboos such as: all the devotees must eschew eating dog and snails as well as avoid sexual intercourse before proceeding to war.[25] These are some of the reasons which account for the localization of the authority of a divinity to a particular socio-political area.

Apart from the war divinities, there are the guardian, prosperity and fertility, and ethical divinities. [26] The ethical divinities abhor stealing, cheating, perjury and other similar vices which militate against societal coherence and stability. Oaths are usually taken in their names and they punish the offenders who falsely swear to them. These divinities, in conjunction with the ancestors, assist in the preservation of the societal morality and ensure harmonious living among the Urhobo. These divinities do not act on their whims and caprices but depend on *Oghene*.

In addition to their above functions, the *edjo* and *erha* are also believed to reveal efficacious medicine to their devotees in dreams. Pa Eyitemi expressed this same view in my interviews with him. He asserted that the origin of medicine could be traced to the divinities which revealed medicines and their specific instructions and taboos to their votaries. These medicines, he opined, were later shown to relatives with the same instructions. But peculiar to Urhobo is that, the owner must put sand on the hand of the person he is/was showing the medicine. The meaning of this ritual act is that he has not hidden anything as regards the medicine; and it also symbolizes that wherever this medicine is used, it should be efficacious. It also shows the granting of the right to use the medicine. It therefore acts as entering into a convenant with the person. Thus, the Urhobo solicit their assistance in order to achieve a happy life. In the praxis of traditional medicine, such divinities which reveal efficacious medicine are invoked by the medicine men.

Erivwi-Ancestors

Erivwi applies to the cult of *esemo* (fathers of children) and *iniemo* (mothers of children). The Urhobo believe that there is another realm of existence after death. Death is, therefore, viewed as a transition to the other realm. It is this belief among Africans that made Mbiti designate the ancestors as the "living-dead". In Africa, in spite of the transition of the ancestors, they are believed to be still living in the spirit world and actively participating in the affairs of their families and are zealously watching the conduct and activities of the living members of their families.

The ambivalent role of the ancestors in the Urhobo belief system that the living-dead bless the living with children, health and wealth and at the same time punish those whose behaviours amount to the infraction of family morality and disruption of the harmonious interaction and co-existence among the living is well brought out. Such misdemeanours include stealing, cheating, adultery by a wife, incest, witchcraft, sorcery and other vices perpetrated especially within the family. The ancestors expect the living to adhere strictly to the laws and moral code they handed down to them. Among the Urhobo, the perpetrators of these vices are regarded as sick persons who need healing.

A deceased member of a family (a living-dead) becomes paterfamilias, an ancestor when the heir has performed the second burial rites and from that point of time the paterfamilias can mention his name when praying to the *esemo* and *iniemo*, the ancestral fold.[27] Among the Urhobo, this accounts for the importance attached to second burial ceremonies and how extravagantly executed. To become an ancestor, one needs to have a child (or children) who will perform the second burial ceremonies, and "ensure the continuity of the individual (father of the child) as the child is seen as the externalization of the father's personal immortality,"[28] a concept which enforces polygamy among the Urhobo. In accordance with this concept, Mbiti asserts:

> Unless a person has close relatives to remember him when he has physically died, then he is nobody and simply vanishes out of human existence like a flame when it is extinguished. Therefore, it is a duty both religious and ontological, for everyone to get married; and if a man has no children, or only daughters, he finds another wife so that through her, children (or sons) may be born who would survive him and keep him (with the other living-dead of the family) in personal immortality.[29]

The ancestors having passed into the spirit world are no longer limited by time and space. They are the better intermediaries (than the divinities) between *Oghene* and *ohwo* (man) in consequence of having passed through *akpo* (physical world) with all its associated problems. Now imbued with supernatural power, the ancestors can bless, preserve and sustain the family in a whole and healthy state and punish by plucking away the nefarious in his youthful days. [30] The libation poured and food given to the *esemo* and *iniemo* (ancestors) are in Urhobo belief symbols of fellowship, communion and remembrance. Mbiti sees them as "mystical ties that bind the living-dead to their surviving relatives". [31] The worship of the *iniemo* and *esemo* (mothers of children and fathers of children) is a regular religious ritual among the Urhobo. Writing on the worship of the *iniemo*, Bradbury remarks:

> The *iniemo* are also worshipped in most cases by the women. They are served during annual festivals and whenever circumstance demanded. Offerings are made in the middle of the compound or on a veranda by the senior woman of the family lineage. A married woman (to the family) does not take part in her husband's *iniemo* rites except her own *iniemo*. [32]

The religious Urhobo, solicit the assistance of the *esemo* and *iniemo* in all their undertakings, be it farming, fishing, business, marriage, medicine-making, *et cetera* as handed down by their forebears. Although the composition of reality in Urhobo worldview seems to be dual, there is, however, a single terrestial cognition with functional attributes from both existence; the two worlds are harmoniously integrated.

The Urhobo believe that the universe is basically good with the great forces constantly at work struggling to maintain a greater unity of all life forms. Man can only achieve what he is capable of, if he co-operates with these forces. It is against this background that in Urhobo, man does not find fulfilment as an individual but as one who participates in a family and community. This is what S.U. Erivwo describes as "a being-in-relation", a peculiar quality which makes man not to be in relation with other beings of the same species but with *Oghene, edjo* and *erha* [33] Relationships, therefore, with other people is of vital importance. The Urhobo understanding of relationship between the individual, family, members of the extended family and community is clearly brought out by Mbiti's statement, "I am because we are, therefore, I am". Nyang pursuing the African concept of the good relationship further argues that it is the need to maintain good relationship between God and man, man and other elements in the universe and man and man that has led to an ontological emphasis in African world of social values. [34]

Troubles of all kinds are related to breakdown in human relationships. And the well-being of everybody hinges on the preservation and restoration of these broken relationships. Worship becomes the vehicle for concretizing this symbiotic relationship between man and the spiritual forces in which each party has to fulfil its own obligation. The inability of man to fulfil his own obligation creates an imbalance in his total well-being which will consequently lead to disorientation if appropriate step is not taken in time to remedy it. Conversely, the Urhoboman does not hesitate to show the divinity the tree with which it is made, if it proves ineffective. This disorientation might be physical, psychological or spiritual. Thus, the state of well-being or wholeness in the Urhobo context goes more than mere physical fitness but wholeness experienced in the rapport with nature, in psychic and social integration in the world of cosmic forces and the level of human morality. [35]

The Urhobo believe that life is man's greatest gift from God and it, therefore, belongs to Him. All efforts are geared towards restoring, strengthening and preserving it. The African concept of man as image *Dei* presupposes a deliberate and concerted effort to preserve, restore and enhance life. [36] The taking of life even in war involves serious sanction. As Placid Tempel rightly points out: "Life belongs to God. It is He who summons it into being, strengthens and preserves it". [37] The Ashanti's belief that when God brings illness he also provides medicine to cure it, [38] corroborates Tempel's remark. Medicine is one means of preserving, strengthening and enhancing life.

In traditional medicine, living is as religious as the cultural background is religious. Healing is also religious and it includes the use of incantations, rituals, divination and medicine; the combination of which remedies the physical and/or spiritual sickness that led to the disorientation of the chemical equilibrium of life. In Urhobo worldview, disease is not only attributed to forces in the spiritual realm but also associated with the preternatural forces in the social world. Such forces include witchcraft, sorcery, breaking of taboos or breaking relationship with a neighbour. This evinces that the Urhobo worldview is religious since the Urhobo is described as deeply religious.

Arthur Leonards's remarks that the Africans eat religiously, drink religiously, bathe religiously and dress religiously [39] is apposite. This portrays the pervasiveness of religion in Urhobo life. The Urhobo worldview is based on the fundamental belief on which hinges all aspects of life. There is a definite course and place for all activities, inventions and events in the world order. This finally became manifest as religious beliefs and practices which underscore the treatment modalities of traditional healers.

From the analysis of the Urhobo cosmology, it is pertinent to conclude that the Urhobo cosmology is an alive universe as Rattray also remarks in his empathetic study of the Ashanti religion and culture. The Urhobo cosmology is indeed viable and maintains an effective social order. [40]

A COMPARISON OF URHOBO AND WESTERN SCIENTIFIC COSMOLOGIES

The Urhobo cosmology differs from the western cosmology basically in its concepts of *oke* and *ophephe* (time and space), *edjo and erhan* divinities and the ancestors as agents of affliction and disease and in the Urhobo concept of man and his environment. The concept of *oke* (time) is of vital significance not only to those in the traditional societies but also to those in modern societies.

The concept also serves as a key to the understanding of the basic Urhobo religious and philosophical concepts. [41]

Concept of Time

Generally, the African concept of time (the Urhobo not an exemptional) has been a subject of very serious disputation among scholars. The main thrust is the African perception of the distant future, whether it exists or not in the minds of the Africans. Some Africans, out of nationalistic verve, contend that Africans conceive time as the westerners whose time moves from the past through the present and to the future. Others maintain that Africans pay no attention to the chronometric recknoning of time. [42] Arising from the various points of view, it is definite that African concept of time differs from the western. Mbiti, for instance, posits that Africans conceive time as a two-dimensional phenomenon, having a long past, a present and gradually tapering future. He contends that African concept of time is contradistinguished from the western: that the westerners think of theirs in a continuum or linear form with an indefinite past, present and infinite future, but that in the African concept of time, the future is attenuated because "events which lie in it have not taken place, they have not been realized and cannot, therefore, consist time". [43]

Mbiti's concept of time has been severely criticised by scholars of African philosophy and culture. Kwame Gyekye is specifically annoyed with Mbiti's assumption that Africans have no concept of the distant future. Basing his argument on his research among the Akan of Ghana, he demonstrated the contrary. Gyekye views Mbiti's generalization as being dangerous because he failed to get a word for the future among the two East African languages he investigated. Based on the Akan concept of the Supreme Being, Gyekye asserts: "The fact that Onyame dwells in an infinite time gives the lie to the supposition made by Mbiti that Africans do not have a concept of a long or infinite future, for surely a concept of an eternal, infinite implies a concept of infinite time." [44]

Sulayman Nyang, on the other hand, only accepts Mbiti's conceptual scheme in so far as it aids the understanding of the particularism of African thoughts. He, however, objects to Mbiti's classification of time for being too simplistic [45] and argues that Africans have a present, a past and a future. He sees the difference in the African's inability to limit himself to the unilinearity of history and believes that this is essentially the difference between African and western concepts of time and space. [46] The western concept of time is diagrammatically illustrated thus:

Past   Present   Future

Animalu conceives the western scientific cosmology as emanating from the

Judeo-Christian religious tradition which indicates life in a linear creation axiom that views the world as "irreversible and undimensional, moving along on an imaginary straight line from a genuine beginning to some definite goal,"[47] while the African worldview (which forms part of the Urhobo), is described as curvilinear axiom of immortal regenerative cycle which Wole Soyinka represents in his poem as "creation snake spawn tail in mouth". As Soyinka puts it: "As the First Boulder, as the errant wheel of the death chariot, as the creation snake spawn tail in mouth, wind chisels and rain pastes, rust from steel and bones, wake dormant seeds and suspended lives". [48]

The African concept of time is cyclic corresponding with the agricultural seasons. Instead of the western numerical calendar, Africans have a phenomenon calendar in which the events or phenomena constituting time are closely related to one another as they occur. Hence Kalu remarks: "Time is peopled with events related to the movements of the sun, moon, important events, in the lives of the family, clan and village-group and socio-economic events such as market days etc. It is never abstract". [49]

Among the Urhobo, time is reckoned by events. For instance, the year begins with *oke ra 'kekako* (planting season), *oke ro rho* (harvesting season) *oke ro ore* (festival season) and *oke ro whe* (flood season). Thus the death of a man, birth of a child and when Mr. A came home from Lagos and so on, are intimately related to and reckoned by these events. [50] This time reckoning is similar to what Mircea Eliade described among the non-complex societies based on what he designated as Myth of Eternal Return. It is based on how the seasons of the year repeat in an eternal cycle; this, the non-complex societies perceive as the eternal order which governs the universe. [51]

Concept of Space

The Urhobo like the African concept of space is problematic. There are three dimensions of space: *odjuvwu* (sky) is where the Supreme Being and the major divinities inhabit; *akpo* (earth) is the abode of *ohwo* (human beings), patron spirits of human activities, nature spirit, earth goddess and ecology while *evuoto* (underneath the earth) is inhabited by evil spirits like those of bad deaths, and those who lived bad lives while on earth, others who did not receive their second burial ceremonies, *oji* spirits and so on. This compartmentalization of the dimensions of space does not mean that each operates on its own. All are so well integrated and intertwined that functionally they operate as one and any attempt to render them asunder distorts the whole. It is in realization of the tight interwoveness of all the aspects of life of the African who is described as incurably religious that Professor K.O. Dike observed:

> Africa in particular, has confronted scholars with communal societies
> where science cannot be separated from religion or religion from law

and politics; where history is nothing but the history of the whole culture, a seamless garment of such fine-woven texture that attempts to separate single strands merely distorts the whole.[52]

The western scientific cosmology which derives from the Judeo-Christian religious tradition also has three dimensions of space; viz: heaven, earth and the underworld. Heaven is depicted as the throne of God and the angels; earth the abode of men and other principalities and powers, and the underworld the abode of the dead. However, the western scientific cosmology emphasizes the visible universe as its area of operation. The African cosmology requires that good relationship should be maintained with the malignant forces and the supernatural forces. To achieve this, worship and taboos are designed so that man can achieve the good things of life.

Conclusively, the Urhobo (African) concept of time evinces the world as moving externally in regenerative cycle of birth, death and rebirth (reincarnation). It is on account of this that it is described as cyclical and irreversible but reckon with a biologically impressed clock. The western concept of time views the world as moving along imaginary straight line with a definite beginning towards some definite goal. It is thus reversible, linear and measured by a mechanically externally impressed clock. [53] A. O. Anya summarizes the African cosmology thus:

> Most African societies, including the Nigerian society, operate on a cosmological framework in which time is conceived as cyclical and space is organized in three compartments: the heaven above, the earth below it and the underworld beneath the earth — all conceived as contiguous and continuous, once more in a cyclical continuum. [54]

Origin of Man

Zoologically, the origin of man is traced within the context of primate evolution especially as humans share a common progenitor with the living representatives of the ape family of primates. However, until 1859 when Charles Darwin published his book — *The Origin of Species,* the biblical belief in the creation of man was still current. By the time the attack and counterattack on Darwin had settled, it became accepted that humans like other animals evolved in keeping with the evolutionary theory. This conclusion was reached due to the essential similarities between the anthropoid apes and man. Some anatomical and behavioural characteristics are shared by both. This is the western scientific concept of man.[55]

In Urhobo belief system as well as other religions, this evolutionary theory of the origin of man is greatly questioned. The way Darwin was attacked and criticised by the Church attested to this. As in Christianity, the Urhobo believe that man was created by the Supreme Being. Mythical stories abound in Africa which relate the creation of man. Essentially, the Yoruba creation myth is a paradigm. The myth has it that *Olodumare* delegated authority of moulding lifeless man of a peculiar shape, look and colour to His archdivinity, *Orisa-nla,* while the prerogative to give life (breath of life) was reserved by *Olodumare.* The Urhobo tell theirs in a similar way but in it, the uniqueness of *Oghene* is emphasized. The details of man's creation are not emphasized. It is said that man moulded a lifeless man to which man could not give breath of life. All man's attempts were to no avail. In man's perplexity, *Oghene* came, told man to back him after which *Oghene* breathed on it and the moulded man became a living being. [56] Thus, the uniqueness of God's creative capability is emphasized.

The Urhobo view man as constituted of *ugboma* (body), *enwe* (breath or heart) and *erhi* (soul or spirit). [57] *Enwe* (breath or heart) is man's intangible and indestructible soul which Brandon describes as "a non-physical entity in human nature". [58] G. E. Okeke describes the soul as something in man which is incorruptible and departs body at death. [59]

Generally, Africans believe that man is made up of his body (soma), personality soul (psyche) and spirit or the motivating breath of life (pneuma). The Christian's view of man's constituent parts corroborates the African concept. The body comprises the instincts of the flesh, eyes and the pride of life. These are what Paul in Galatians Chapter 5 verse 19 called the works of the flesh which include: fornication, impurity, licentiousness, idolatry, sorcery, enmity, strife, jealousy, anger, selfishness, dissension, party spirit, envy, drunkenness, carousing and others. The mind or soul is made of the intellect, the will and the basic personality structure, while the spirit, Paul describes as portraying the fruit of love, joy, peace, patience, kindness, goodness, faithfulness, gentleness and self-control (Gal. 5: 22 & 23). In western cosmology, man is viewed as a biological being while in Urhobo (Africa), man is a biospiritual being. This accounts for the variance in both medical practices, in the concept of life and the means of restoring, preserving and enhancing life or health.

Western orthodox medicine is based on Graeco-Western science model with its emphasis on empirical verification of evidence. Disease and sickness are explained biologically and bacteriologically. This indicates that disease and sickness are due to malfunctioning of the human organs arising from the action of certain bacteria and counteraction of some chemicals in the body. Disease is thus viewed as a physical disorder. Anatomic operation and physiology are viewed as the only means of discovering the ultimate secret of human life form. All bodily events — good health, illness and mental function have to conform to the anatomic and physiological processes.

Medical expert, by mutually combining the results of the different tests and observations can diagnose diseases and prescribe their cure without reference to supernatural causative agents. As a cosmology built on empirical verification of evidence, it is guided by a body of explicit acceptance/rejection criteria which ensures the efficiency of science. [60] This is why western orthodox medical practice concerns itself essentially with pathological state without emphasizing the wholeness of man. Although cases of psychosomatic and psychiatric diseases do exist, the influence of the environment as a potent causative factor was not considered.

In Urhobo cosmology, the three components of man — the body, soul and spirit affect the well-being of one another. Disease or sickness is attributed to natural/physical, spiritual, socio-psychological and moral causations. The African cosmology is religious with the different modes of existence well integrated. This is why in the case of sickness, the diviner is consulted to ascertain the root cause of sickness, and to recommend appropriate remedy or rituals to perform. In some cases, the medicine man takes care of both the physical and spiritual aspects of the diseased state; thus ensuring the wholeness of his patient. In most cases, more than one causal factor may be involved. There are no criteria that determine mono-causal or multidimensional causal origin of sickness. It is the diviner who reveals this during the divination process. Thus, healing is a continuous productive process which involves all aspects of life. As Iwu rightly points out:

> Healing is not to be viewed as lifeless product but as a production. Not as an act that ends with the administration of remedies but an activity that includes all aspects of living. It presents itself to us as the continual recurring work of spirit, not as a finished and final product. [61]

However, in orthodox medicine, the role of external influences which do not originate from the brain or other parts of the body, are not accommodated. This point does not deny the existence of esoteric science among the Europeans but the argument is that it is not incorporated into the orthodox medical system.

Africans believe that the Creator imbues both animate and inanimate objects with life forces. It is this life force which the objects have imbibed that connects them. This life force is the quintessence of the thing itself. This includes man, trees, beasts, or stone. This life force in the object is only properly harnessed and used by the knowledgeable and the initiated. Often, a medicine man talks to a tree, animal or stone in the course of his profession. He is not appealing to the organic property of the tree, herb or the stone but he is appealing to the life force. This he harnesses and uses for the benefit of his patient.

This attitude of the traditional healer was misconstrued by foreigners to mean animism. Here the medicine man is not worshipping the spirit or life force of the phenomenon but rather appealing to it for the benefit of his patient. In Urhobo religion, everything exists because of man. This underscores the supremacy of life and centrality of man. Hence, Urhobo religious attitude to life is world-affirming and described as anthropocentric. This is one of the few points on which Mbiti and P'Bitek have a common agreement. As Booth (Jr.) remarks: Mbiti and P'Bitek, who disagree on many other things, agree that in Africa, God or the gods seem to exist for man". [62]

In traditional medicine, any treatment that does not focus on the multi-dimensional causations of sickness is greatly frowned at. Traditional medicine as vehicle for restoring wholeness and enhancement of life is more than the use of roots, leaves, barks, fruits, grasses, insects, bones, shell, feathers, powder and other objects in the preparation of medicine. Medicine-making involves herbal medicine, psychotherapeutic, spiritual and socio-moral healing techniques, Metuh also supports this point, and views medicine-making as encompassing herbal mixtures, magical objects, rites, incantations capable of affecting change for better or worse. [63]

In traditional medicine, the roles of the ancestors, divinities and the spirits are significant for its efficacy. If a patient is given a decoction to drink or bathe with, he not only has faith in the life force in the leaf or the active principle of the *materia medica*, but also considers the role of the ancestors, the benevolent gods and spirits in realizing the cure of the diseased state. In Urhobo, disease is intimately related to these spiritual agents and its cause is meticulously diagnosed before treatment. The Urhobo perception of the causation of disease and its treatment derive from that appreciation of their cosmology which is essentially religious. Una Maclean points to the involvement of the cosmic agents in sickness and its treatment thus:

> The African demands an explanation for the particularity of the individual misfortune. Such an explanation may be afforded by the belief in witchcraft, by faith in the power of magic, by recognition of forces controlled by the gods or set in motion by man, by a whole range of ritual observed or disregarded. [64]

Apart from the deities, ancestors, and spirits, disease is also attributed to psychic agents like witchcraft, sorcery, an evil-eye, curse of ill-willed member of the family, the deviation from the norms of morality, or social relationship by the individual or members of his family or the whole group. It is noteworthy that among these malevolent and malignant agents of affliction, it is the pervasive influence of witchcraft that is still widely acknowledged. This does in no way negate the Urhobo belief in natural causation of disease but in most cases external forces are blamed for stubborn and protracted disease and death. Invariably, various diseases demand various therapeutic modalities — medicinal, psychological, magical rituals and so on.

In all cultures, man is the centre-piece of all the cultural phenomena. Culture has been defined as an abstraction which encompasses the total way of life of a society. It is the precipitate of a group expressing its adaptation to the physical environment. [65] Briefly defined, culture is the totality of man's way of life. In nearly all creation myths, other creatures are depicted as emanating from God or from the creative functions he delegated to his functionaries, but with no other creature had God an intimate relationship as with man. The Genesis myth tends to support the supremacy of life. It evinces life as the spark of God in man — "Let us create man in our own image". The supremacy of life and the centrality of man in the context of the African ontology has earned Afrel a title and thus described as *anthropocentric. Anthropos* derives from Greek which means man; while *centric* means centred around. This indicates that Afrel is centred around man. Thus the gods and other beings exist because of man; yet man depends on the whims of these capricious gods to accomplish and realize his full capacity in life. Therefore man lives a precarious life. [66] The Genesis story is more definite and piquant when God Himself said "Let him (man) have dominion over the fish of the sea and over the birds of the air, and over the cattle, and over every creeping thing that creeps upon the earth". [67]

The Urhobo believe that life is man's greatest gift from *Oghene* and it therefore belongs to Him. All efforts are geared towards its maintenance, preservation, restoration, and enhancement. War is a means of expressing man's instinctive tendency of self-preservation when life is threatened by external aggression. That serious sanctions are still attached to its elimination attests to its primacy. [68]

In all cultures and among all peoples of the world, the preservation of life is uppermost. Man in the course of his daily life, preserves life through the consumption of diverse food items that appeal to him. Man discovered to his astonishment that in spite of all his efforts to preserve life, it is still subjected to acts of diminishment. God perhaps foresaw this that He directed man to eat all the plants and fruits on the earth to counteract the effects of the various diminutive agents. [69] The origin of religion, magic and science has been traced to the series of attempts made by man to placate, manipulate and control the supernatural beings in order to harness and utilize all available forces for his well-being. However, religion opposes magic and science because of its fundamental assumption that the supernatural beings control nature and human life. Hence, religion tries to gain the favour of these beings through sacrifices and prayers. Magic, on the other hand, compels such forces of nature to its wishes through the sheer force of spells and enchantments; science, fundamentally, controls these supernatural beings through mechanical pressure. It has been contended that the failure of magic led to the development of religion. [70]

In the course of the eating of plants and fruits, man discovered that some had therapeutic properties. Thus the provenance of medicine is traced to the process of trial and error experience. Man's experimental use of plants is distinct from that of the animals for it would have been difficult for man to differentiate good therapeutics from the multifarious materials available. [71] Man was, however, guided by some outstanding characteristics such as peculiarities of taste and smell. Usually medicinal plants are pungent, bitter, aromatic and astringent. These qualities narrowed down the choice of herbs for the practice of trial and error. [72] Medicine was discovered in this way as a means of preserving and restoring life whenever it falls into a state of discomfort, disease and ill-health. People all over the world developed and thus have different ways of preserving and curing diseases. [73] These can be discussed under the following:

(i) Health;

(ii) Disease; and

(iii) Healing.

Health

The World Health Organization in 1946 defined health as a state of complete physical, mental and social well-being and not merely the absence of disease or infirmity. [74] Rothschub, on the other hand, defines health as a state of feeling well in the body, mind and spirit, together with a sense of reserved power, based upon the principles of healthy living, a harmonious adjustment to the environment (physical and psychological); it is a means to a richer life in service. [75] Health, therefore, involves the integration of the physical, spiritual and the psychosocial elements in man. Health is the primary concern of the Urhobo. Health is preferable to wealth. Hence, the Urhobo say *oma kpokpo ne efe and ufuoma ne efe*. The Urhoboman would rather suffer and remain in abject poverty in order to maintain and live a positive and sustained state of health. The Urhobo say *oma kpokpo oya ose r'ohwo* (Health is man's lover). This, the Urhobo say because a healthy man is an asset to his community. He will not only contribute meaningfully to the development and growth of the society but also keep the societal laws and regulations. Conversely, a sickly person retards progress and accelerates societal insecurity and deprivations. This is why the Urhobo, like every other African, leaves no stone unturned to seek and acquire health.

Disease

The definition of disease is fraught with many difficulties consequent on the standpoint and purpose of its usage. Thus, various philosophical, metaphysical, anthropological and religious schools, psychosomatic medicine, social medicine, health, politics, doctors and patients define it from their perspectives. Rothschub in defining disease from man's perspective sees it as "a subject and/or clinical and/or social need for help, which is based on a loss of tuned cooperation of physical, psychic or psychophysical functional elements of the organism" [76] He argues that in the disease, there is functional disturbance where harmony is replaced by contradiction and cooperation by discordance. The symptoms were due to the change or extinguishing of the regulatory processes in quantity or quality. In addition, the Urhobo consider afflictions and the breaking of the moral code as disease.

Healing

Healing is the means of restoring by curing sickness. Rothschub defines healing as an act of regaining the cooperation of all the functional elements in the organism.[77] Healing, in the Urhobo context, comprehends more than mere curing of sickness. It is the restoration of the wholeness of man physically, psychologically, spiritually, mentally, psychically and socially. This contrasts the western concept of healing which means merely the restoration of only the pathological state. Thus, disease, in the Urhobo context, is not only a disequilibration of body balance causing physical discomfort but also a slump in a man's business, difficulty in securing job, a partner for marriage, and so on. Generally, disease or illness is universally anxiety provoking . Man's process of life could be diagrammatically represented with a triangle.

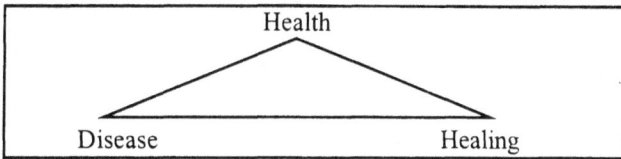

```
                        Health




          Disease                      Healing
```

Man has a vital force, like every other phenomenon created by God, known as *Vis Medicatrix Natura* (the healing power of nature) which constantly strives to maintain and sustain the wholeness of the body. [78] This vital force may be overpowered by both internal and external agents of diminution and consequently a state of disequilibration of the balance of the body systems leading to discomfort and ill-health. The state of ill–health (or causes of disease and sickness) is interpreted variously by different people depending on their perception of their cosmology.

The western scientific cosmology attributes the cause of diseases and sickness to the germ theory, which postulates that all diseases and sickness are due to the activities of bacteria and the malfunctioning of some of the biological and chemical reaction in the body. This theory claims that diseases are caused by deadly micro-organisms. It holds that to destroy these micro-organisms requires the discovery of another germ or antitoxin, which will wage war against them and annihilate them. Thus drugs of very high potencies are compounded and used to kill germs found in the human body. Such drugs capable of destroying micro-organism in the body can also be injurious to the living cells.[79] This, scientific cosmology evinces man as a biological being. Thus, the aetiological explanation of diseases and sickness is derivable from the biological and bacteriological perspectives without reference to supernatural causation.

The Urhobo cosmology, which undergirds their perception of disease, differs immensely from the western scientific cosmology. Invariably this will, no doubt, dictate their causal explanation of disease and sickness. Healing in the Urhobo context does'not limit itself to the restoration and preservation of the disequilibration of body balance causing physical discomfort. It includes healing of slump in business, inability to achieve one's aspiration which causes discomfort and disease in social relations. Therefore, illness includes:

(a) disease; and

(b) afflictions.

Disease, sickness and pain are universals. All cultures have developed different healing processes to cater for these universals. However, the interpretation of these universals is dictated by the cosmology of the people. Consequently, there is an intrinsic relationship between the practice of medicine and culture. In consonance with this view, W.S. Mensah-Dapa vouches that "not all diseases in Ghana are due to bacteria, viruses, spirochaetes, parasites, malignant tumours or nutritional deficiency. There are ailments in Ghana whose root cause can be found in witchcraft and juju"[80] Johannes Aagaard similarly opines that "behind the vast offering of health and greater comfort, you find a distinct worldview determining the basic concepts behind alternative healing."[81]

It is in consonance with this view that scholars of a different hue, including Mensah-Dapa, argue that there are ailments which occur as a result of our traditional environment of mystical or spiritual causation, and that these can only be cured by purely local medicines. Ademuwagun has argued pungently that "It is an established fact in medical care that no realistic health personnel can reasonably disregard or minimize the importance of cultural equation of health, sickness, disease and medicine."[82]

In the light of the foregoing, the praxis of western medicine also has limited value in other cultures. Payer's comparison of the practical application of western medicine in industrialized countries of France, West Germany, the United States and England, is educative and informative. These are countries with equivalent life expectancy rate, yet, Payer discovered great differences, which reflected the differences in cultural background.[83]

TAXONOMY A: TYPES AND CAUSES OF DISEASES

The aetiology in traditional medicine is categorized into three main dimensional factors. These are: natural or non-supernatural, psychiatric and social or preternatural, and supernatural causation.

Natural or Non-Supernatural Diseases

The Urhobo recognize that there are natural diseases which emanate from the inability of the organic systems to function adequately. This attestation authenticates the relevance of such questions as *Worie-emu none re?* (Have you eaten today?) or *Wo neri none re?* (Have you gone to toilet today?), whenever a man complains of headache, bellyache and so on. Natural or non-supernatural diseases include: *uyovwimiavwo* (headache), *oworhe* (catarrh), *orakpara* (cough), *ekpromose* (ring-worms), *unusoroyoro* (haemorrhoids pile), *usuoma* (dysentery), *oraevu* (stomach ulcer), *uyovwirobie* (giddiness), *edja* (worms), *edjarame* (guinea worm), *ekpae ve omamiavwo* (fever), *ekpae* (cold), *ugbere* (gonorrhoea) and so on.

Natural diseases are usually caused by the disequilibration of the bodily chemicals. However, naturally caused disease which fails to yield to the whole gamut of proven efficacious therapy is consigned to supernatural causation. This is based on the Urhobo belief that naturally caused diseases are fertile grounds for agencies of supernaturally and psychiatric/socially/preternaturally caused diseases to operate. Thus Byaruhanga remarks that the failure of physical remedies prescribed for treating empirical ailment enables people to believe that witchcraft or bad magic is at the background and it is apposite. [84] The Yoruba, on the other hand, believe that preternatural agents could cause or worsen natural or physical ailment. [85]

Social or Preternatural Diseases

Social or preternatural and supernatural diseases are more involving and are usually in the cultic realm. Social/preternatural diseases are extremely refractory to normal therapeutic treatment whose efficacy is proved. In addition, the treatment may involve sacrifice. In most cases, recourse is to psychometry, to discover and ferret the cause of the ailment. Ayoade sees the characteristics of a preternatural/supernatural disease in its being "severe, chronic or exotic... but the resistance of an ailment only indicates the possibility of a supernatural cause. Thus, the diagnosis of such a preternatural/supernatural ailment follows the recital of its history which is fed into the diviner's board". [86]

Social or preternatural diseases emanate from the activities of witches, sorcerers and evil eyes of enemies. Witches are believed to possess inherent powers with which they nocturnally prey on human souls. Their activities are not only directed towards an enemy but also to friends, relatives and parents out of jealousy. Their activities are so inimical and anti-social that in Urhobo most illnesses and deaths are associated with them. Parrinder remarks that "as the witches devour the "spiritual body", so the mortal frame weakens. Its blood is sucked away spiritually. Pains, paralysis or impotence appear different members." [87] This is also the belief of the Urhobo.

They do not utilize any physically concocted herbal preparation. Rather, the forces inherent in nature are at their disposal for manipulation to their own advantage. This is the major point of departure from sorcery, which in general parlance is bad magic. Sorcerers, therefore, possess magical preparations with trajectory powers capable of harming somebody aimed at from a distance.

Supernatural Diseases

Supernatural diseases are mainly due to breakdown in relationship between the ancestors and their progeny, breaking of taboos and committing offences against the divinities. This broken relationship, in most part, arises from children's dereliction in their filial obligations towards the ancestors, [88] failure to accord a befitting second burial and breaking of family morality. On the other hand, divinities are believed to bring an erring votary to answer for his/her deviant behaviour from the accepted norms and their failure to fulfil their votive obligations. In fact, any person who commits an abominable act, hated by the divinities, ancestors and men, is regarded as sick in Urhobo. Such abominable acts include adultery committed by a wife, incest, murder, stealing of yam, goat, etc. especially those of a priest-family head, a priest of a family divinity or a priest of a village divinity. As the *Ovie* (King) of Ogbara puts it: "Incest is a very serious taboo and it is rarely broken but when it is broken, the consequences are always grave." [89]

In this case, the traditional specialist who performs the healing of a sick soul is the *Orhere* (priest). He has to perform sacrifices of propitiation to the ancestors and/or divinities. Thus in the divine ministration of both the priest and the votaries, they must keep themselves ritually pollution free and things must be done in the way they were handed down to them.

Special Remark

The preternatural/supernatural causation of diseases is a belief, which constitutes a metaphysical article of faith among the Urhobo. This is why Gelfand with his wealth of experience in traditional medicine warns orthodox doctors who practise in Africa to be better acquainted with the aspects of African life which have medical bearing. [90] This metaphysical article of faith is subjective truths accepted by the Urhobo and regarded as objective truths. W. Z. Concu views the problem of communication between traditional and orthodox medical systems as essentially emanating from this. Hence he remarks that:

> The problem of communication between traditional and modern medicine essentially concerns the divergence of subjective truths accepted by African believers and regarded by them as objective truths. Thus the truths of faith and the truths of science resemble one another in social consequences, though they differ in the method of demonstration, proof or verification. [91]

The preternatural/supernatural causation of diseases, the Urhobo believe, explains all complexes of extraordinary diseases. To the Urhobo, this is true and they are psychologically convinced even though conclusive empirical backing cannot be adduced. It is a truth that cannot be falsified empirically or verified but some of its claims are factual. These factual claims are existentially determinative based on the experience of the Urhobo during the process of acculturation. However, there are basic regional differences. As Gelfand records, "running throughout all researches, we notice a basic pattern and a basic philosophy. It is obvious that the traditional African believes first that disease is caused by a spirit or supernatural agency, and secondly that many illnesses can be alleviated or even cured by the administration of one of the many remedies found in nature.[92]

TAXONOMY B: TYPES OF THERAPY

The aetiology in traditional medicine as classed above warrants different medication. As has been mentioned above, the supernaturally caused diseases require psychometry to ferret the root cause. The available therapeutic methods adopted in traditional medicine of the Urhobo are basically eight. Mume noted that Nigeria has the highest variety of therapies and that this has placed Nigerian traditional medicine in a superior position to other countries. [93]

Umwu (Herbalism)

It is the treatment of ailment through the use of herbs. Herbs and other vegetable remedies form about 90%; hence the name herbalists. [94] In some cases, parts of animals, insects and so on may be included. Herbalism is the oldest form of therapy. Its origin is coeval with the evolution of mankind. It was used by the ancient Egyptians, Greeks, Chinese and Romans. It is believed that Hippocrates, the father of medicine, employed herbal remedies in his treatment of ailments. Even the Bible also affirms the use of herbal remedies. For instance, God said to Adam "from every tree in the garden, you must eat to satisfaction". The use of herbs is universal and Nigeria has many herbalists of high repute.

Urhobo herbal medicines display some mystical forces. For instance; there are some that possess occultic strength, some are *ifue* (antidote) which counteract disease supernaturally caused, some *umu-use* can be telepathically directed to summon a missing person, a run-away, from distance, *oyoreghono* or *oyoriwe* assist in the extraction of bullets or thorns from the body without any surgical operation. *Ekpofia* is used to divert bullets from the target person or spot, mere chewing of *umuokpo* renders the user invulnerable to enemy's attack. The enemy cannot raise his hand up to fight the user while *umuora* or *umu ri sie ihori ne ora* is a natural antiseptic which fights against microbes in the body. Herbal antiseptics not only heal the body but also assist in building up new cells.

There has been a call to move from the use of synthetic drugs to galenical treatment and the use of herbal medicine. This has assisted in proving that African medicinal plants and their remedies are efficacious. This current movement has consequently led to the study of African medicinal plants.

Eghworo (Massage)

The Izon whose environment does not permit the growth of many herbs specialize in massaging. This therapeutic system has been employed for the treatment of ailment of the nervous, muscular and osseous system. It is specially used for treating gynaecological problems. The whole armamentarium of the masseur is the physical manipulation of the muscles, joints and veins on the nude skin in a technical manner. In most cases, massage treatment may be applied to relax the muscles and veins, and to allow circulation of blood. Massage aids the stimulation of muscles, joints and veins and allows circulation of blood.

The therapeutic method has spread to the contiguous neighbours of the Izon: the Urhobo, the Isoko and the Itsekiri. The inability of the Izon to produce herbalists of high repute is the function of the nature of their environment which does not permit the growth of sufficient vegetation.

The Greeks also made use of massage therapy and today massaging has been employed by German and Swedish physicians as scientific treatment. It is based on the physiology and anatomy of the human body.

Ame vwo nyoma (Hydrotherapy)

Amevwonyoma implies the application of water of different forms and temperature for the treatment of ailments. Its curative value is realized by both the practitioner and those who have gone through such treatment. Its curative effect has been discovered of late by scientists.

By equalizing the circulation of the blood in all the systems of the body, hydrotherapy aids in increasing muscular tone and nerve force, improving nutrition and digestion, thereby increasing the activity of the respiratory glands. Hydrotherapy facilitates the elimination of broken down tissue cells and poisonous matter and other noxious issues which impinge on the proper functioning of the body systems.

Hydrotherapy involves the use of cold, hot, compressed and steam vapour baths. Cold and hot baths are used for the treatment of different diseases after the addition of some herbs. The fusion is then used for fever, headache, rheumatism and general pains. The hot bath not only makes the skin capillaries relax but also increases the activity of the sweat glands. It has been discovered that water increases the consumption of oxygen to about 75%; while about 85% of the carbon dioxide in the body is eliminated through the use and consumption of water.

The compressed bath comprises a piece of cloth wrung out of cold or hot water which is applied to some part of the body to produce the desired temperature. Hot fomentation is specially useful in the treatment of ailment such as pains, soreness, inflammation, rheumatic troubles and swellings, among others. Traditional midwives use hot fomentation for newly delivered mothers to relieve pain, relax the muscles and to allow the distended muscles of the stomach assume their normal position.

Ohwevwechiro (Fasting)

Ohwevwechiro as a means of cure for some ailments was realized from the early history of man. Domestic animals are known to fast for days to enable them recover early from an ailment. Although the beneficial aspects of fasting might not be obvious to the traditional medical practitioners, they adopt it in their therapeutic system. It is used mostly for the treatment of *evurokere* (constipation, indigestion), *ekpevu* (obesity) and its related diseases. It is also useful in the treatment of spiritual diseases.

Eating too much without corresponding exercise and proper elimination of the waste results in overloading and overworking of the body systems; it slows down the process of digestion and elimination; eventually producing a condition known as auto-intoxication or self-poisoning. Autointoxication is the underlying cause of some acute diseases. Fasting, in a situation like this, yields good results within a short time and the most effective means of eliminating such waste. Mume describes fasting as:

> The most effective means of body house-cleaning known. Fasting is an eliminator of accumulated toxin as well as a general restorative. Fasting is a purifying process. It brings about a rapid elimination of toxic and poisonous materials from the body.[95]

Traditional medical practitioners often prescribe fasting before drinking some concoction. This mode of treatment might continue for many days until the ailment is completely cured.

Uboemuo/Egho (Cupping or Blood-letting)

This form of therapy is extensively used in Nigeria. It was effectively adopted in the African and orient civilizations. It is the method of abstracting impure blood by the use of the abstraction cups or horns. In Northern Nigeria, the horn has long been used for blood-letting. The Urhobo call it *Uboemuo* or *Egho* and it is regarded as an effective treatment for rheumatism and other morbid condition of the blood. The Indians appreciate blood-letting as a means of sustaining good health. It is one of the best antiphlogistic measures. During the Victorian Medicine, it was recommended by Simpson, Professor of Midwifery, as a measure for reducing placenta congestion and inflammation. As he puts it, "General blood-letting, repeated or not, according to circumstances, along with more or fewer other antiphlogistic measure, has been long successfully employed... (this enquiry shows) the value and rational character of this practice."[96]

The therapy has metamorphosed from lip-suction cup and horn to cupping instrument, which was discovered by Junod in the middle of the 19th Century.

Since then, this therapy has been used by orthodox medical practitioners in many parts of the world.

Laboratory experiments have confirmed the adequacy of this therapy. For instance, they have indicated that cupping gives rise to positive changes in the white blood corpuscles, the alteration of the sedimentation rate of the context of the serum and the concentration of the hydrogenous and the formation of active histamine bodies; this helps to decrease the congestion rate in the tissues. Histamine effects this through the dilation of the veins.

Blood-letting was initially condemned seriously but today its positive function has been acclaimed. It is effectively used in traditional medicine.

Oma evuvwo (Heat Therapy)

Heat therapy is significant in traditional medicine or healing system. Tradomedicalists have recognized the potency of the vibration emanating from fire. Fire is a vibratory force. Harmonious vibration of the body cells means good health, discordant vibration of the body cells results in disease, while the seizure of the vibration of the body cells results in death.

Sun and fire are sources of energy. Treatment derived from sun-rays is known as *heliotherapy* while that derived from the light and heat of fire is known as heat therapy. The utilization of heat therapy by traditional healers has resulted in the successful treatment of acute and chronic diseases, since it aids in the maintenance of better condition of health. Fire light or rays have the quality of increasing metabolism in the tissues of the organism by penetrating deep into the body thereby creating lethal condition for bacteria, relieving pain and increasing the rate of oxygen consumption. Consequently, it leads to the modification of body tissues.[97] The beneficial functions of fire healing is achieved by the removal of accumulated impurities through the many pores of the skin. Any delay in the removal of the accumulated impurities results in autointoxication or self-poisoning.

In Urhobo medicine, heat therapy is effected by preparing a fire with logs and when the smoke has reduced and the charcoals are burning brightly, the patient is required to expose the affected part of the body to the direct rays of the fire. In some cases, clothing materials are removed from the body and the patient either lies or sleeps beside the fire. This assists in calming down nerves and regulating muscular contractions and adequate circulation thus inducing sound sleep. This method is perhaps one of the reasons our forebears lived up to ripe age (80 to 140 years).

Mume asserts that high blood pressure, stomach ulcers, kidney damage, diabetes and liver malfunction which take the largest death toll in modern generation were not common among our forebears and rural dwellers of the present generation. He attributes their low rate of incidence to the fact that the people lived according to natural laws that govern life. [98]

Omebere (Surgery)

Urhobo traditional medical practitioners are adepts in the performance of intricate operation to remove bullets and poisonous arrows from wounded tribal fighters. They operate on the belly to extricate noxious tissues which cause unnecessary disturbance and stitch it together by technical application of pieces of calabash on the operated part while the sore gradually heals.

There are traditional anaesthetic drugs which are applied to the operated centre to subdue the pains partially or completely before the performance of the operation. The drugs are mainly herbal mixed with oil after it has been reduced to paste. This preparation is applied overnight. The Urhobo call such medicine *umuedri*. Unfortunately, the custodians of this therapy are gradually dying off and the remaining have become too old to continue the science.

Esivwo re esegbuyota (Faith Healing)

In traditional medicine, faith healing is one of the therapies. In Urhobo, it is associated with medico-religious practice. In the ancestral cult, the patient who commits a sin against members of the family and is being tortured by the ancestors, is made to confess his sin. After the confession, the patient is relieved emotionally after he has been pronounced forgiven. This also is the function of sacrifice in the African traditional medicine. Sacrifice helps to relieve the patient of all his emotional worries which might be the underlying cause of the disease. Ezebasili perceives the understanding of African medicine not only in knowing the therapeutics but "also a good knowledge of the dynamics of the culture, especially the importance of sacrifice — the crucial psychological point of all cults and an essential bond between man and deity." [99] Professor Lambo, a well-known authority in psychiatry, has also attested to the therapeutic function of sacrifice.

Another means through which faith healing is achieved is through *Igbeuku*. This cult plays a significant role in Urhobo medicine. It is robbing herbalists of many clients. Members of this cult are forbidden the use of any herbal or orthodox medicine. Their emphasis is on faith and the application of native chalk *(orhe)* in the treatment of diseases. [100] *Igbeuku*, faith therapy, is beneficial in treating psychologically and emotionally induced ailments. Its armamentarium includes the use of incantations and prayers together with vigorous dancing which is a guilt-reducing exercise. This situation makes for effective treatment of anxiety, inferiority complex, suspicion, fault-finding and others. *Igbeuku* claims authority over wizard-and-witch-induced disease, demon possession, and sinful ones whose guilty conscience tortures everyday. *Igbeuku* compares favourably with all the shades of Christian healing ministries whose emphasis is also on faith healing. Faith is the bedrock for the acceptance and appropriation of the power of Jesus. As Jesus commands the apostles: If you had faith as a grain of mustard seed, you could say to this sycamore tree, "Be rooted up, and be planted in the sea", and it would obey you. (Lk. 17:6).

The various therapies that exist in Urhobo medicine have linkage with other cultural medicine. Some of the therapies have been scientifically developed in other parts of the world and introduced into orthodox medicine. Mume has asserted that Nigeria has more numbers of therapy than other countries of the world. Nigeria, therefore, is capable of developing her own medical system. The problem with Nigeria is that we have been so brain– washed by the missionaries and British colonial government to the extent that Nigerian government and people hate everything Nigerian. They painted the natives as a sort of quintessence of evil. They are regarded as "insensible to ethics; they represent not only the absence of values, but also the negation of values. They are the enemy of values, and in this sense, they are the absolute evil".[101] The attitude of many Urhobo (Africans) towards their cultural values and heritage has been very negative.

The attitude of the government towards traditional medicine has been discouragingly backed by the orthodox doctors who view the traditional practitioners as rivals. However, since 1980 in accordance with the World Health Organization declaration that local materials and personnel should be utilized for the local health delivery system of the people, government has changed its attitude. But a place of prominence has not yet been accorded it. There are some laws which do not give free hand to the practitioners of traditional medicine.

TAXONOMY C: TYPES OF MEDICINE

The classification of traditional medicine depends on the use each culture puts it into. Among the Urhobo, medicine is not classified into male and female as Anthony U. Uzoma has identified among the Igbo. However, it is sickness which is so categorized. Hence you have, male and female measles, chicken pox, stroke, hypertension and so on, corresponding to their severity and how the disease responds to treatment. Thus, the attack of chicken pox, small pox or any other which is easily cured or treated, is regarded as *iphori* (female) while that which is stubborn is regarded as *oroshare* (male). To some extent, *iphori* (female disease) corresponds to natural disease and *oroshare* (male disease) corresponds to preternatural/supernatural diseases. Urhobo medicine is classified into four categories viz: therapeutic, love and life enhancement, protective and destructive.

Therapeutic Medicine

Urhobo medicine is primarily for healing disease and the restoration of wholeness to man. Wholeness refers to restoring the physical, the psychological, the spiritual and societal moral order. Evil is disruptive to the ontological harmony and sickness or disease is the symptom of such evil. With the assistance of the medicine man and/or diviner, the cause of the patient's diseased state is discovered through the diagnostic methodology. In such cases, the restoration of wholeness may involve knowing sacrifices and other rituals, to be performed which must be preceded by herbal treatment based on the cause and nature of the disease. The sacrifice and other rituals will restore the ontological order of the society where the ancestors, divinities, witches and sorcerers are involved. Thus, the cosmic harmony is restored. As J.V. Taylor argues:

> A man's well-being consists rather in keeping in harmony with the cosmic totality. When things go well with him, he knows he is at peace with the scheme of things, and there can be no greater good than that. If things go wrong, then somewhere he has fallen out of step. He feels lost. The totality has become hostile, and if he has run out of bad luck, he falls prey to acute insecurity and anxiety. The whole system of divination exists to help him discover the point at which the harmony has been broken.[102]

Magical Preparations: Good magic

Magic is categorized into two: good and bad. The Urhobo call good magic *umwu/uhuvwu* which is used to the advantage of the individual or society. On the other hand, bad magic often designated as *orha* (sorcery) is used to cause misfortunes, diseases and so on to the detriment of man or society.

Magical Preparation for Love and Life Enhancement

The success of every marriage depends on how the husband and wife/wives sustain the love that prompted them into the marriage contract. However, because of one domestic problem or the other, the love is mitigated and the husband or wife flirts. In most cases, women find it difficult to sustain their husband's love. Hence both literate and illiterate men and women, but especially women, resort to making *inewheri* (love magic) from medicine men. This is an attempt to keep together the household by reducing to minimal unchaste attitude. The phenomenon is clearly demonstrated in *The Concubine* by Elechi Amadi when Wonuma, the mother of Ahurole, Ekweme's wife, advises her daughter to make a love potion which will bind her husband securely to her so that Ekweme will forget Ihuoma, his lover. Some love preparations have side effects which in most cases render active and intelligent husbands passive, stupid and dependent as Anyika explained to Ahurole.[103]

There are other magical preparations which improve the luck of some people who find it difficult to get a job, wife or husband and improve their business. This is a kind of love magic which helps to sweeten one's relationship with others. My informant indicated that the materials for preparing such medicine include granulated sugar, soap, sponge, water and centipede. The patient performs a ritual of whirling the centipede round his head seven times at a cross-road while saying "anything that prevents me from getting a job should be removed from me". At the end of the seventh time, he buries the centipede at the intersection of the roads. After this, he goes to the river for ritual cleansing. He washes with the sugar, soap and sponge from his head to toe while saying "as from now all my relationships with all people should be as sweet as the sugar." Anything that makes it difficult for me to pass any interview should be cleansed away and let my relationships be as sweet as sugar." [104] The medicine is mostly used by people who find it extremely difficult to pass interviews, or get a wife or a husband. This mystical preparation brings out the Urhobo philosophy that life could be made unpleasant for others by evil forces like witches, sorcerers or evil eyes of enemies.

Protective and Life Enhancement Magical Preparation

Man is constantly haunted by the fear of insecurity arising from the hostile environment in which he finds himself. This sense of insecurity does not only emanate from malignant forces but also from man and events like road and fire accidents, gun shot and cutlass. Consequently, people go to medicine men to prepare medicines and charms that prevent, or protect them from such attacks.

In an environment where witches and sorcerers dominate, women often go to medicine men for preventive medicine against abortion during pregnancy and other types of medicine which ward off evil spirits or forces that prevent them from being pregnant or destroy newly conceived children in the womb. John Munonye portrays the Igbo belief in this aspect in his book, *Obi*. Emenike, the medicine man gave Anna, the barren woman, a leather belt to wear around her waist to prevent evil spirits from destroying her seeds of life. [105] In the traditional Urhobo community, a woman who aborts during early pregnancy often wears *edaji* (meaning "stay") [106]

Protective amulets are worn by children around their neck, waist or hand, while others have incisions in the body against poison and paediatric diseases, convulsion, measles, snake bite, knife-cut, gun shot, sorcerers, witches and other evil forces. According to Ezeanya: "There are many cases of charms which medicine men tie and put on the neck or waist of children and even adults either to cure a particular stubborn disease or make them immune to it. [107] Magical preparation for protection assists in obtaining promotion in one's place of work, to win popularity and to sustain it, promotes one's business and enhances life generally. Hunters need protective medicine to guide them against animal attack, attack by evil spirits and from being harmed by their own bullets. In court cases, protective medicines are often worn by the defendants and plaintiffs to secure favourable judgement from the judge. Judges also wear them for protection against attack. In some villages, one often finds bundles of charms (*egbo*) tied at the outskirts. These are mystical preparations for protection against epidemics like small pox and other evil forces that might be sent to it by her rival village or witches or sorcerers. They are, in most cases, prepared in rings, incised in the body, prepared in small bags worn by individuals.

Munonye reports that among the Ibagwa people, many of the government workers wear charms or magical preparations on their bodies for promotion or protection in spite of their being Christians.[108] Even today, both Christians and Moslems are strongly attached to the use of protective medicine.

Orha (Sorcery)
Destructive Mystical Preparations

These are the most feared medicines. Evil people and sorcerers often employ them at the least provocation. Sorcery functions essentially to bring illness, misfortune, failure and death to those at whom it is directed. The medicine man and people who practise sorcery are often feared.

The individual may be harmed by putting the poison in his food. Isidore Okpewho, in his book *The Victims,* describes how Nwabunor eventually caused the death of her mate, Ogugua, her three children and Ubaka, Nwabunor's only son through the poison she procured from Eze Nwozomudo. This destructive medicine was performed through contact with the individual or the food items, drinks and other chewables.[109]

Destructive medicine operates mostly from a distance without any physical contact. It involves the projection of the mind and the victim is abstracted and appears before the operator of the sorcery. Whatever is done to the abstracted image or the effigy of the victim is believed to happen in the same way and intensity to the physical person. It operates with the principle of similarity. The sorcery cannot be effective without the use of the words of intention or incantations. Munonye describes how Ozigbo, the medicine man, through the use of sorcery attacked Jumbo, Sam's opponent thus:

> The snake that bites stone must lose its fangs, he said and picked up his metal staff. He that seeks to destroy others must be prepared to be destroyed himself. He watched the bare ground silently, with great concentration. Then he took a cool, steady aim. He stabbed. The metallic thud almost shook the ground. He's here, he proclaimed and held the man — whoever it was — there, at the point of the staff for about a minute. Not long after, some subdued rumours began to spread. Jumbo had pitched backward, he dropped down, foaming at the mouth.[110]

Orha (Witchcraft)

It is the most potent, destructive agency in the Urhobo traditional society. Its activities are so anti-social and inimical to the growth and development of any society; all untoward occurrences are attributed to it. In most Urhobo societies, the activities of *erieda* (witches) are directed to their family members. Hence, among the Urhobo there are sayings like *oruwevwi-ruohwo ohwo ro rie ohwo oye rue ohwo* (it is the person who knows man that bewitches him). *Uwevwi da rhovwe k'ohwo ko yere omamo akpo* (if one's house/family agrees for one to live good life then one can become prosperous) The corollary is that if an Urhobo man struggles to live a prosperous life but in spite of it all he could not make it; the Urhobo say *uwevwi roye rhovwe ke-e* (his family does not agree with him). These are subtle and trenchant references to the nefarious activities of witches. Gelfand remarks that ancestors remove their protection if the relationship is strained. In such a case, witches can operate successfully.[111] Gelfand's remarks corroborates the interview I had with Chief Atuya on the seriousness of the sanction placed on the committal of incest in Urhobo. Chief Atuya of Okpara Waterside remarks:

Wo de ruemu re erivwi nu,

Esemo ve iniemo ki siobo ne ohwo na,

ko nerhe kemu kemu ebraba efa ke phia ke.

When a person offends the ancestors,

the ancestors withdraw their protection from him. And

anything evil can now happen to him.[112]

P. A. Dopamu holds witches responsible for all family misfortunes. As he contends: "Witches are held responsible for illness, death, sterility, ill-luck, unsuccessful harvest. In fact, all misfortunes which occur in the family and the whole villages are attributed to witches.[113]

In all its usage, witchcraft connotes the destructive employment of mystical power. This is how Mbiti[114] and Parrinder[115] describe it. Specifically, Mbiti defines it as a "term used more popularly and broadly to describe all sorts of evil employment of mystical power, generally in a secret fashion while Parrinder uses it to designate harmful employment of mystical power in all its different manifestations. The Urhobo designate this destructive and aggressive element of their traditional medicine *orha;* and it is referred to throughout Africa as African science or black power. For instance, Olusegun Obasanjo (twice Head of State) once advocated the employment of black power to dismantle the oppressive apartheid regime in South Africa.[116] Oguakwa and Animalu made similar remarks.

However, among the Urhobo, witches are classified into two categories.

(1) a wizard/witch who uses his/her power in healing and generally for the good of the society is known as *Adjene* (celebrated witch who had confessed his/her sins and resolved to do good). In most cases, *adjene* are *ebo* (medicine men) while

(2) *Orieda* is a witch who resolves to do evil and whose activities are mainly executed during nocturnal operations. [117]

CHAPTER THREE

Diagnosis and Treatment

INTRODUCTION

In chapter two, it was argued that the understanding of the Urhobo cosmology is the open sesame to understanding Urhobo medicine. Based on this, three factors that could cause disease have been identified and incidentally these are also the types of disease among the Urhobo. Thus there are natural, social/preternatural and supernatural diseases. The diagnosis and treatment of diseases are intimately related to the people's perception of disease. As it has been argued, the Urhobo cosmology is essentially religious. Thus in the treatment modalities, *egophiyo* (incantations) and rituals are many since the supernatural forces especially the *esemo* and *iniemo* — fathers and mothers of children (ancestors) — must be invoked to ensure the efficacy of the treatment. However, the diagnosis and treatment of natural diseases do not involve the employment of *egophiyo* and rituals except those at the peripheral level.

These *egophiyo* will be examined in the context of the Christian Healing Ministry. This will, no doubt, aid the understanding of the utilization of *egophiyo* in different contexts. Rituals will also be investigated in the same way. But it is argued that some rituals are intrinsic while others are extrinsic in Urhobo medicine. The role of the Urhobo medical practitioner is also examined. Finally, the chapter argues that rituals are effective vehicle for effecting treatment of preternatural and supernatural diseases.

NATURAL DISEASES

Natural diseases are diagnosed mainly through its symptomatology. The Urhobo traditional medical practitioner does not only depend on the symptom but also takes the history of the diseases, examines the whole body especially the affected area, the eyes, the temperature of the body so as to determine whether the patient is strong or weak. This will assist the healer to know the type and quantity of medicine to give to the patient.[1]

The treatment and prevention of natural diseases are effected through the application and administration of medicament whose toxic qualities could be verified in a laboratory test. Its treatment is rational because it is within the domain of herbalism.

Natural diseases are usually caused by the disequilibration of the body chemicals or injuries sustained physically. However, natural disease which fails to yield to the whole gamut of proven efficacious therapy is consigned to supernatural or mystical causation. This is based on the Urhobo belief that natural diseases are fertile grounds for agencies of supernatural and social/ preternatural diseases to operate.

My interviews have revealed that the collection, preparation and administration of medicine for natural (physical/physiological) disease (that is the treatment) do not involve many rituals and incantations except those at the peripheral level. For instance, a very efficacious medicine for arthritis which Mr. Eyarunu Eyimofe of Ugono-Abraka refused to divulge was prepared for my wife who could not sleep for three nights after hospital treatment. During the collection of the *materia medica*, the preparation and administration of the remedy on one ritual was observed or performed even though Mr. Eyimofe continued to assure me of its effectiveness. My wife who was in gruelling pains took the concoction and in less than thirty minutes, the pains had subsided. Today my wife is cured of the arthritis which is described in medical books as stubborn.

Mr. Odiru Omorohwovo, a renowned osteopathist at Eboh-Orogun handles orthopaedic cases without any serious ritual and invocation of the ancestors. In his treatment of fracture, Mr. Onorohwovo breaks the leg of a hen and ties the patient's and hen's legs with the medicine after he had thoroughly massaged and put the broken bones in their proper position. As the hen's leg heals so also the patient's leg heals. Mr. Odiru Onorohwovo claimed that the day the hen walks properly, the patient would also walk.[2] However, the breaking and treating of the hen's leg with the medicine is a form of ritual which affects the psychological state of the patient.

An effective medicine for natural waist pain is seven lobes of alligator pepper, camwood and the bone of the waist of a hen or cock. All the lobes and the waist of the hen/cock are ground to powdery form and mixed with native drink *ogogoro*. It is administered by lacerating the patient's waist and rubbing the paste onto it. My informant[3] attested to the efficacy of this medicine and gave names of those he had treated successfully with it. To ascertain the authenticity of the claim, I interviewed some of the people who confirmed the assertion.[4] However, Una Maclean has questioned the need for the use of number of items as "seven" in the above medicine. She feels that the number might have some magical effect. This accounts for her designation of such medicine and treatment as magico-rational.

The attachment of magical or mystical effect to number is not peculiar to the Urhobo medical practitioners. Among the Euro-American mystics, the number 'thirteen' arouses their apprehension. As common as sky-scrappers are in the western societies, it is alleged that thirteen-storey buildings are rare. It was this same mystical and superstitious belief that made my colleague, Dr. B.J.E. Itsueli indicate his preference for Room 14 instead of Room 13 initially allocated to him as office.[5] However, among the Urhobo generally, including their medical practitioners, there is preference for *ese* (odd) and not *odi* (even) numbers. Numbers one, three, five, seven, nine and so on are significant in Urhobo traditional medicine.

Traditional doctors Aje, Onorhime and Chief Akpojivi attributed their significance to the ancestors who revealed such medicine to their progeny. They claimed that failure to adhere to the numbers renders the medicine ineffective. But S. N. Enunuaye explained the mystical signification of some of the numbers thus: '9' represents maturity, perpetuity and irreversibility and '3' stability and reliability. Thus, before a traditional medical practitioner administers a remedy or passes the knowledge of medicine to a patient, he makes sure that he counts up to nine while he puts some sand in the patient's palm and says: *Ose ke we or Ose ghorowe* (may the medicine be efficacious for you). The import of this is that the traditional medical practitioner or whoever prepares or has the medicine, has wholeheartedly revealed the secret behind the medicine to the person. Once this is done, the medicine retains its potency at all times. The sand indicates that he has not hidden anything from the patient or the person who is acquiring the medicine. The fact that Urhobo medical knowledge is, for the most part, experiential and not experimental, is well brought out because this was how the ancestors jealously did it.

It must, however, be noted that every culture has its disposition towards certain numbers and these affect the people's inner state, self-image and their relationship with others. In Urhobo medical system, the therapeutic scope of ritual depends on how it affects the patient's inner state, self -image and his relationship with others.

Medicinal plants used by traditional medical practitioners have been discovered to be effective in cases of hepatitis, fractured bones, malaria, ulcers, intestinal hurry, convulsion and hypertension. Earache, eye troubles, headaches, and cold are treated with herbal preparations applied as eye or nose drops. Sore, muscular complaints and various veins are treated with smears of herbal preparations. Internal diseases are usually treated with drinks prepared from herbs, barks and roots. Impotence in man is handled with preparation mixed with some preparations from herbs, roots and barks. On the whole, in natural diseases, the services of psychometrists are not required.

PSYCHIATRIC/SOCIAL/PRETERNATURAL AND SUPERNATURAL DISEASES

In the treatment of social/preternatural and supernatural diseases, there are various *egophiyo* (incantations) and rituals. During the diagnosis, recourse is had to psychometry to pry into the cause. These categories of diseases are characterized by seriousness, elusiveness and refractoriness to the whole gamut of proven efficacious therapy and are usually inexplicable. It is then the duty of the *Oboepha* (diviner) to determine the right course of action to be adopted to ensure effective cure. During the process of divination, there is direct communication with the unknown. Divination affords the *Oboepha* the means of predicting the future or discovering the cause of some inexplicable events in the past. This desire to comprehend the unknown is universal among humans. However, its frequency is determined by the economic and social stability of the group. Humans always turn to some form of support during period of uncertainty or stress situation especially to religion which provides spiritual and psychological security [6]. A diviner scarcely diagnoses diseases being naturally caused. His thinking is that the patient's relatives would not have bothered to consult him if the ailment had not proved stubborn. Hence, diviners usually graft on some supernatural factors. This, no doubt, gives psychological satisfaction to the patient and the relatives. In consonance with this assertion, S.U. Erivwo remarks: "Only the *Oboepha* (diviner) can say the actual cause of death. He would generally not be expected to say, and would never say that it was natural" [7] Z. A. Ademuwagun has identified two main types of diagnosis:

> (i) Disease-centred diagnosis: Here the focus is on the diseases or some other disturbances which impedes proper bodily function, explicable in terms of knowledge of anatomy, physiology or pathology. The process involves history taking, observation and clinical test. This type of diagnosis is applicable only to western medical practice.

> (ii) Person-centered diagnosis: This relates to the practice of traditional medicine. The reasoning behind it is that the treatment of any disease involves the physical, social and emotional/psychological management of patients. [8]

Ademuwagun argues that the traditional medical diagnosis and treatment are more intricate, brilliant and effective methods of dealing with the total person of the patient. In addition, the relevance of a patient's personal and sociocultural beliefs, values and practices as they relate to his expectations, needs and interests are also examined. Thus, the diviner is consulted to ensure the rendering of maximum help to the patients in their interaction. Hence, Ademuwagun remarks:

> A critical analysis of the diagnostic methods shows that the traditional health personnel are astute and shrewd behavioural scientists of no

mean capacity. As pragmatists in their own profession, their brand of behavioural science is in consonance with sociocultural and psychological situational reality in the patient's total environment.[9]

He, therefore, concludes that the diagnostic approach of the traditional practitioners is indicative of their awareness of psychosomatic disorders and health ecology.

Ayoade has identified a third cause of disease, which he designates as God-sent. The symptom of such a disease is its persistence, resistance to proved medication and its ultimate incurability. Thus AIDS according to his argument could be so classified. However Mume, a tradomedicalist denies the incurability of any disease. He describes disease as the desecration and breaking of natural laws which regulate both our lives and health. He views disease as the consequence of our trespasses against the natural rules of health. As he remarks:

> With every disorder suffered by human being, tradomedical method of treatment can provide a cure, provided the patient is willing to adopt the traditional and normal methods of treatment embodied in tradomedicalism.[10]

He further contends that traditional medicine as a distinct, separate and comprehensive healing system for preventing and curing disorders and abnormalities caters for the whole being.

The causes of diseases, diagnosis and medication may be diagrammatically represented thus:

Types of Illness	Causes	Diagnosis	Medication	Result
Disease	Non-supernatural	Observation and experience	Therapeutic manipulation	Cure effected
Affliction	Anthropomorphic supernatural (Caused by man's evocation of the spirit)	Observation and experience / Resistance to proven rational treatment divination	Therapeutic manipulation and ritual purification	Cure effected
Supernatural	Divine (caused by God, divinities, spirits, ancestors)	Observation and experience / Resistance to proven rational treatment divination	Therapeutic manipulation and ritual purification	Cure may be effected or not

*Diagrammatical Representation of Diseases, Diagnosis and Medication **Ayoade**, 1979.*

CURATIVE AND PREVENTIVE MEDICINE

Rational Treatment

From the taxonomy of traditional medicine, the causes of disease in Urhobo medicine is classified into three: viz. Natural/physical: social/preternatural or mystical; and supernatural. Involved in the diagnosis is the healer's knowledge of both the causes and classification of illness. Thus, the diagnosis of natural disease is effectively performed through a systematic questioning and the physical examination of the patient. In some cases, the traditional practitioner asks for its history and carefully listens to what the patient says. The history usually entails the patient's description of the disease, how it developed and the various steps taken so far to cure it. From the history, the healer gathers more details about the symptoms, location of the disease and its exact form; thereafter, he undertakes further physical examination of the patient. As I have mentioned above, rational treatment of natural disease does not involve many rituals. Below are some examples of natural diseases and their remedies.

DISEASE, *MATERIA MEDICA*, PREPARATION AND ADMINISTRATION

Abortion 1-3 Months (Prevention and Treatment)
Ishakpa seeds (*Jathropha*) cray fish, potash, native pot (*emevwere*) salt.
Grind seeds and cray-fish together and boil. Add potash and salt to taste.
Drink as pepper soup.

Bleeding during Pregnancy

Awolowo leaves (slam weed or *eupatorium odoratum*)
Wash neatly and extract liquid.
Drink one glassful of the liquid.

Nose Bleeding or Ordinary Bleeding

Eran (ocimum basilicum) leaves.
Squeeze leaves to produce liquid.
Put liquid in/on the affected part.

Nose Bleeding

Ebe ikpamaku (African marigold).
Squeeze leaves to produce liquid
Put in the bleeding nostril while patient faces up.

Chest Pain

1. *Oghriki* (new *bouldia lewis*) seven leaves, *erhie* (alligator pepper), as many seeds as possible.
    Chew the leaves and alligator pepper together.
    Spray item on the chest.

2. *Arhua* leaves (seven).
    Chew the leaves thoroughly.
    Spray front and back of chest. Spray remnant into air facing the sun in the east.

3. *Ebe uzo* (antelope) leaves (seven), Ripe plantain.
    Wash neatly.
    Chew items together while saying the following incantation:
    Uzo muo oga-a (seven times) (antelope does not get sick).
    Repeat for seven days.

4. *Oghriki* (new *bouldia lewis*) bark, kolanut with three lobes, mortar, carapace (tortoise back).
    Grind bark in a mortar, smoothly pack it inside the tortoise back and put kolanut on top.

    Before washing mouth in the morning, pack bark in mouth; chew a lobe of kolanut together and spray on the chest and later on the wall. Do this for three days.

Stomachache, Constipation, Indigestion

Lime fruit, (*Otie ogagan*). Squeeze out juice and mix with *ukehu* (potash). Drink mixture; patient belches; positive reaction noticed after 30 minutes.

Constipation and Indigestion

Ohahe (Silk cotton tree-*Caibe pentendra*) - leaves.
Extract liquid.
Drink infusion.

Prenatal Treatment of Convulsion

Wall-geckos, (seven-dried) salt.
Grind dried wall-geckos and add salt, add pomade.
Put drops in mouth, eyes, centre of head, two toes, and two thumbs.

Convulsion Treatment

Obaekpe native pomade.
Squeeze leaves and pomade.
Put drops in mouth, eyes, centre of head, two toes, and two thumbs.

Another Convulsion Treatment

Native pomade, fire soot.
Mix items, together.
Apply into the eye of the child.

Cough

1. *Ameme,* seven leaves, *erhie* (alligator pepper), seven seeds.
   Chew items together.
   Spray the chest.

2. *Eti*-the flowers, plantain (one seed), salt, oil.
   Grind *eti* flowers in a mortar, add oil and salt to taste. Roast plantain.
   Use the roasted plantain to eat the paste.

3. *Obe Okpokpa* (*Bryophillum*)- leaves, salt.
   Roast slightly; squeeze out water and salt to taste.
   Drink for seven days.

Diarrhoea

Ode (plantain) sap, food
Mix sap with food.
Eat.

Difficulty in Breathing during Pregnancy

Okpagha (oil bean tree), seven leaves, alligator pepper (seven seeds).
Chew items together.
Spray on patient's chest and stomach.

Ubrenwen (Difficulty in Breathing)

Ugboduma, leaves and stems, spices, oil.
Grind items together, add oil and boil.
Rub on all the body. It produces immediate cure.

Driving away Snakes from Infested Area

Bitter Kola.
Put as many as possible around the place.

Dysentery

Oruru (cotton-*Gossypium arboreum*) leaves and flowers.
Extract liquid from leaves and flower and drink.

Earache

Ode (plantain) sap from inflorescence.
Collect sap from inflorescence.
Use as eardrop

Eczema

1. *Ebeevwe* leaves (*Macabus scraba*) and kerosine.
   Squeeze as many leaves as possible together, and add kerosine.
   Rub on affected parts. Healing takes place 48 hours later.

2. *Amoke* leaves
   Squeeze as many leaves as possible together
   Rub on affected part.

Eczema and Ringworm

Uwara tree (latex), red sand.
Scrape the affected part with sand and collect latex.
Rub latex on the scraped part.

Elephantiasis

Eke (African wood oil-nut tree: *Ricinodendron.*
Africanum) bark.
Pound bark and mix with water.
Apply on affected area.

Ero re ibigho kpare (Eyes with Cataract)

Oze, ebe re ikpe meku erha (three), native pomade.
Squeeze items together. Add pomade.
Drop liquid as eye drops in the morning and evening.

Evuerhorho (Heat in the Womb during Pregnancy)

Ishasha, Akata - (roots) *urierie*, water.
Grind items together and add water.
Drink infusion.

Evuorhorho (Heat in the Womb during Pregnancy)

Owo re uzo (weed), *irhiboto, owo ru uzo* (leg of the animal).
Cray fish (seven), one pepper cut into seven pieces, salt and native salt.
Grind all items and boil, add salt and native salt to taste.
Drink three times a day.

Eye Trouble

Agogo (crab wood-*carape procera*) bark.
Reduce bark to powder, mix with water.
Use in washing eyes.

Fever

Egberebo root.
Wash and boil. Put items into a bottle, add *ogogoro*.
Drink decoction.

Fever and Headache

1. *Arhua*- seven leaves, chew.
    Spray it on the head.
2. Pawpaw leaves as many as possible, palm wine, sugar or salt,
    Squeeze all items together in palm wine, drink.
3. Pawpaw seeds (as many as possible), cray fish, spices and salt to taste.
    Grind items together and boil.
    Drink as pepper soup.

Fever (Malaria)

1. Pawpaw (ripe fruit).
    Peel and eat.
2. Lemon grassroots.
    Bottle roots, add *ogogoro* or gin.
    Drink.

Fever, Beriberi, Stomachache, Feverish chill

Eto (pawpaw-*Carica papaya*) leaves.
Boil leaves.
Drink decoction.

Flow of Breast Milk

Eto (pawpaw), *latex*, water.
Mix items together.
Wash breast of nursing mother.

Gonorrhoea

Ishakpa roots (Jathropha), *ukehu* (potash).
Put in a pot, add water and boil. When boiling, add potash.
Drink decoction, one glass four times a day.

Chronic Gonorrhoea (Venereal Disease)

Ishakpa roots (Jathropha), *ukehu* (potash), *ogogoro*.
Put roots in a bottle, and *ukehu* and pour *ogogoro*. Allow to dilute.
Shake bottle and take one-two glasses every one hour.

Headache

Ameme (seven leaves), *eshasha* (spices).
Tear the seven leaves on patient's head, throw halves in the left hand away.
Chew halves in the right hand together with *eshasha*.
Spray on forehead.

Human Bite

Coconut roots, *eran*, native pomade. Grind dry coconut roots, add native pomade,
put into a pot and heat, squeeze *eran,* dip into hot pomade.
Apply hot formentation on the spot.
Spray ground coconut roots to the spot.

Idjaghroghro (Parotilis or Lockjaws)

Maize — three years old (*Oka Ikperha, aka* (bitter kola).
Chew sufficient seeds, add bitter kola and chew thoroughly.
Spray on the locked jaws first thing in the morning before washing mouth.
Repeat until cure is effected.

Impotency in Man

Erevwereba (white canalily) - leaves, one needle, seven pieces of broken pot picked outside.
Cut seven apexes of leaves; while pounding, put seven pieces of pot in fire to become red-hot. Mix pounded material with water sufficient for patient to drink once. Put the red-hot seven pieces of pot into the mortar.
Drink hot concoction from mortar (not with spoon). Remove needle and pieces of pot and keep safely for further use if necessary, but patient should lick needle both in the morning and evening emphasizing his desire.

Impotence

Akoro roots, *aka* roots/bitter kola, *eshasha* (spices), alligator pepper and *ogogoro*.
Put all roots together. Grind *eshasha* and alligator pepper into a bottle and add *ogogoro*. Shake bottle and take one glassful three-four times and one during bed time.

Jaundice

1. *Akata* (swizzle stick-*rauwolfa vomitoria*)- roots and bark.
    Pound items together and add water.
    Drink concoction as purgative.

2. *Ugboduma* (frankincense) leaves and stems, (pit) *Erhurhu* (rubbish pit).
    Boil leaves and stems together for about one hour.
    Bathe patient with decoction in *erhurhu* (a rubbish pit).

Jaundice with Maniscal Symptom

Akata- roots.
Pound roots and add water.
Drink infusion as sedative to induce several hours' sleep.

Malaria

Mango leaves, pawpaw leaves, fresh lime leaves, guava leaves.
Boil all items together.
Drink the decoction
Steam bathe the body.

Malaria Fever

1   *Okikpobevwerhe*, seven *irierie.*
     Boil all items together.
     Drink some decoction and bathe with others.

2. Pawpaw (remove seeds), lime fruit and bark of pineapple.
Peel all items together and boil properly.
Drink decoction one glass thrice a day.

Malaria Fever Purgative

1. *Okikpobevwerhe, urhurhoko, urierie* (spices).
Squeeze items together, add salt to taste.
Drink infusion.

2. As *enema saponis.* As in malaria fever purgative above for *enema saponis*
Sift infusion.
Put infusion into patient's anus.

Measles and Itching

Oruru (cotton-*Gossypium*) leaves and flower, *Orhe.*
Extract liquid from leaves and flower and mix with *orhe.*
Rub on the body.

Measles and Jaundice

Ifo (water leaf)- leaves.
Collect juice of the leaves.
Drink juice.

Menstrual Pains

Oruru (cotton-*Gossypium*) leaves and flower, *Orhe.*
Extract liquid from leaves and flowers and mix with *orhe.*
Rub on the body.

Migraine (Severe Headache)

Adjuge-roots, one seed of alligator pepper.
Remove sand without washing. Scrape roots into leaf or leaves
Add one seed of alligator pepper (do not grind). Add small quantity of water.
Drop concotion into the eyes as eye drops (very hot as pepper).

Mouth Wash for Smelling Mouth

Ohahe (silk cotton tree-*Ceiba pentendra*)- bark.
Pound bark and mix with water.
Use infusion as mouth wash.

Nose Bleeding

Ebe ikpamaku (African Marigold).
Squeeze leaves to produce liquid.
Put in the bleeding nostril while patient faces up.

Nose Bleeding or Ordinary Bleeding

Eran-(Ocimum basilicum) leaves.
Squeeze leaves to produce liquid.
Put liquid in/on the affected part.

Odo (Yellow Fever)

1. Fruited pumpkin (*umehe, ugu*), long spices (*urierie*).
    Boil items together.
    Drink for six days.

2. Blue (plant)-roots, *ogogoro*, spices (*urierie and ehirhe*).
    Bottle all items.
    Add ogogoro or any hot drink.
    Drink.

3. Blue (plant)- roots, *urierie, ehirhe,* cray fish, pepper, salt to taste.
    Grind all items together and boil.
    Drink as pepper soup.

4. *Agogo, irierie* (spices)- seven.
    Boil items together.
    Drink some, steam bathe body.
    Bathe with water.

5. *Omoke* (seven leaves), lime-leaves, spices (*urierie eshasha* or *ehirhe*).
    Boil items together.
(a) Drink some.
(b) Bathe patient at 4.00 am. in a dust bin. Remove water and whirl it over patient's head and throw away. Patient should not rub palm kernel pomade.

Oedema (Swollen Feet during Pregnancy)

Corn silk (the tassel or silk from an ear of maize).
Boil large quantity with water.
Take one or two glasses three times a day.

Oga r'one Okeremo rhe (Sickle Cell)

Ebelebo leaves, umuhe leaves.
Prepare soup with them.
Eat regularly to provide blood.

Oga re phe (Diabetes)

Egbona r'imitee (usually parasite on rubber, orange or mango trees).
Dry but not exposed to sun (leaves).
Grind to powder or boil dry leaves and drink as tea.

Ogbarhie (Pain during Menstruation)

Urierie (spices) - (one) *ekete re eshasha* (spices) *eko, iso re erawevwi* (rat faeces).
Grind items together, put into bottle and add *ogogoro* or hot drink.
Take one spoonful once a day before menstruation but stop during menstruation.

Okporoyoro/Unusoroyoro (Pile/Haemorrhoids)
Eran, alligator pepper-one seed, palm oil or native pomade (palm kernel).
Squeeze *eran*, grind alligator pepper and *eran* together, boil items together, add oil.
Insert paste into the anus.

Oraro (Dizziness during Pregnancy, Malaria Fever)

Uho or Ufogbu (roots), spices (*eshasha*), *orhe* (native chalk).
Extract root wood and pound, add *eshasha* and *orhe*.
Share quantity into two.
Add native salt (*ughweri*) to one part.
i.) Add water or ogogoro to native salt and drink.
ii.) Rub other part without salt on the eye.

Oso (Swollen Leg because of Sore)

Three years' corn or maize.
Grind items, lacerate affected part.
Rub on affected part.

Oso (Pit Oedema-Swollen Hands and Pressing in)

Oneya (water yam tuber).
Peel yam tuber and collect water.
Rub on affected part.   It itches.

Pains in the Ribs

Eberirhibo, erhie, ichihi re uzo, ushe, irihiboto and *itetebe.*
Chew all items together.
Spray the affected area seven times while saying *orha ye oga re efe* (if it is the poison or sickness of the ribs).

Piles (Haemorrhoids)

Bitter leaves (juice).
Squeeze leaves to produce juice.
Use to press pile and to touch anus, it will draw inside.

Pneumonia

Ebitien (lemon grass), three or four lime fruits, pawpaw leaves and two dried plantain leaves.
Boil items together.
Drink decoction three times a day.

Pregnancy: Inactive Child in Womb

Arhua (seven leaves), and alligator pepper (seven seeds).
Chew items together.
Spray on the womb early in the morning. It itches.

Reduction of Pains during Labour

Eke (African wood oil-nut tree: *Ricinodenoron Africanum*) bark.
Pound bark and mix with water.
Drink infusion.

Reduction of Weight or Size of Child in Womb for Easy Delivery

Emako (pepper fruit) leaves, *eshasha* (spices) as many as possible.
Chew items together.
Spray on the womb area, both front and back.

Removal of Blood Spot in Eye as a Result of Fighting

Ehirhe or *ewo-o* (spices), water.
Grind and add some water.
Use as eye drops.

Removal of Thorns and Bullets

Kola tree- seven foliage leaves, native soap, three old leaves of kola tree.
Grind seven foliage leaves together with native soap.
Put paste on the affected part, put three leaves on it and tie.

Respiratory Complaints and Asthma

Orugbegwa - leaves.
Squeeze fresh leaves and obtain juice.
Drink the juice.

Rheumatism

1. *Urhenoko (*African peach-*Sarcorephalum esculentus)*
    Pound bark and add little water.
    Tie or apply on affected parts.

2   *Mubighokpayovwi* (goat weed) leaves, as many as possible.
    Squeeze leaves and add salt.
    Lick some and rub on affected part.

3. *Imirhe akpata-* flower, *ughweri* (native salt), *orhe* (native chalk),
    ogogoro or hot drink.
    Grind items. Separate into two, bottle one part and add ogogoro.
    Rub other part on affected part after laceration.
    i)   Drink bottled item.
    ii)   Rub on affected part until cure is effected.

4. Coconut roots, *ukehu* (potash), bone of the thigh of chicken,
    native pot.
    Grind roots together, put ground roots in a pot, add water and boil.
    Add potash to taste — infusion red.
    Suck content with bone of fowl until cure is effected.

5. *Ebeitien* (lemon grass) leaves.
    Pound leaves mixed with *orhe* to form paste.
    Apply on affected parts.

Rheumatism Numbness

i.   *Stagnant Type*

Ishasha, native soap, seven alligator pepper seeds.
Grind items together, lacerate spot of pain.
Apply paste to seat of pain and tie. Loosen and remove on the third day.

ii.   *Moving Type*

Native salt (*ukehu*) bark of *emekpeoto*, one pepper, native chalk, *eti* (monkey sugar cane).
Grind items, put inside bottle.
Take two tablespoonfuls two times daily. Patient may take it once daily depending on constitution.

Ringworm

Amoke leaves, kerosine, red sand.
Scrape affected part with the sand to almost bleeding point, squeeze leaves together and add kerosine.
Rub on the affected part. Very efficacious.

Ringworm and Itching

Bitter leaves.
Extract liquid.
Rub on affected part/area.

Scurry and Indigestion

Origbo (bitter leaves)
Extract liquid by squeezing it in water.
Drink infusion.

Severe Running Stomach

Tomatoes (leaves), four or five lobes of kolanut.
Split kolanut and chew one lobe together with tomatoes leaves.
Chew items together and swallow — very efficacious.

Sleeplessness (insomnia)

Aka roots (Swizzle stick-*Rouwolfa vomitoria*).
Boil roots.
Take decoction after cooling, one glassful as a sedative to induce sleep for several hours.

Small Pox and Measles Prevention

Ugege-bulb, *eshasha* (spices), *Imitegbe* - bulb, *orhe* (native chalk), Camwood.
Grind items together and share into two. Add camwood to one part and mix
the second part with *orhe* (kaolin).
Use two hands to collect each part, and rub on the body.

Snake Bite First Aid

Bitter kola.
Scrape with cutlass or any sharp material.
Chew bitter kola and apply on affected part.

Snake Bite Treatment

Utezi- leaves. Get as many as possible.
Boil leaves with palm kernel pomade.
Give patient to lick.

Sores

Two leaves of *Ikpamaku* (African Marigold).
Squeeze leaves to obtain liquid.
Apply liquid on the sore.

Sores, Burns, Rheumatic Pain, Insect Bites, Ringworm, Jigger, Eruptions, Yaws

Agogo (crab wood), bark yellowish sap from stem
Collect the sap and apply on the affected area.

Spleen

Ibe (seven leaves) and alligator pepper (seven seeds).
Tear seven leaves and divide into two on patient's chest.
Throw halves on the left hand away.
Chew halves in the right hand with alligator pepper.
Spray affected part: chest/ribs under diaphragm to be repeated about three
times every day.

Sprain, Bone, and Nerve

Ogbriki (new *bouldia lewis*) -bark, oil, *urierie* (spices).
Pound bark, mix with oil and spice and boil.
Apply paste on affected area and tie for three days.

Stomachache

1. *Ugege-* young leaves, cut as many as possible, yam.
    Boil items together.
    Eat as porridge.

2. *Imirheakpata* - flowers as many as possible, small pepper.
    irhibo vwievwie or *irhibo emephra* (native chalk), salt.
    Grind items, mould, dry and keep.
    Chew small quantity.

Stomachache, Constipation, Indigestion

Lime fruit (*Otie ogangan*).
Squeeze out water and mix with *ukehu* (Potash).
Drink mixture; patient belches, positive reaction noticed after 30 minutes.

Stomachache, Indigestion and Vomiting

Urhenoko (African peach - *Sarcocephelum esculentus*) bark.
Pound bark and mix with water.
Drink infusion.

Stomach Upset

Awolowo leaves (Siam weed-*Eupatorium odoratum*).
Squeeze leaves in water and collect content or chew leaves and swallow liquid.
Take one glass, three times a day.

Stomach Upset/Fever

Iyeke leaves and native drink or gin.
Put leaves in a bottle, add *ogogoro*, leave for two hours.
Shake bottle properly and take one glass, three times a day.

Stopping Abortion

Asakrase (shell weed), seven alligator seeds, *orhe* (native chalk) and one palm kernel.
Chew all items together.
Spray on the tommy.

Stopping of Bleeding in Cuts and Injuries

Ode (plantain), sap from petiole.
Scrape petiole and collect sap.
Apply on the sore.

Stroke or Paralysis

Oghworoma, native soap, urine of youth and stalk of plantain leaf.
Pound *oghwhoroma*, add native soap. Mix items with the urine. Put on fire to
warm, beat one end of plantain stalk.
Use the beaten part of stalk to touch poultice and rub on the affected parts.

Tuberculosis

1. *Ifierhivwi,* alligator pepper-three fruits, sugar, peppermint and
    ogogoro or any hot drink.
    Grind alligator pepper, bottle all items, add ten cubes of sugar and
    ogogoro or any hot drink.
    Drink.

2. *Uriereiewhu*-roots, palm oil.
    Cut roots and dip into oil.
    Chew and swallow sputum.

Turning Eyes

Odjugbe (thorn), cray fish, native pot.
Burn items together in the pot to ashes.
Lick ashes after cooling while saying *ero bie iku-u*
(*eyes never turn cray-fish*) (seven times).

Ubigho Rokpahe Ero (Eye Cataract)

Ugege stem, *arhua* leaf and little salt.
Extract water from *ugege* stem, put in *erhua* leaf and add little salt.
Use as eye drops.

Ubrenwen (Difficulty in Breathing)

Ugboduma, leaves and stems, spices, oil.
Grind items together, add oil and boil.
Rub on all the body. It produces immediate cure.

Ugbere re Uyovwi (Gonorrhoea of the Head)

Ebe re egodi, iruo nya ubiere agha re ame orhe, isene (onwa)
Orodeko ro vwe uyovwi ive.
Put all items in a container with water and squeeze together.
Wash the head with infusion.

Umbilical Cord

Obiokpokpa (Bryophillum) leaves, native pomade and native pot.
Grind leaves, add pomade and heat material in pot.
Apply on the umbilical cord.

Umbilical Cord

Urierie (spices), native pomade, native pot and a clean piece of cloth.
Grind spices, add pomade and warm paste in pot.
Tie item in a piece of cloth.
Use to press the navel/cord at least three to four times a day.

Yaws and Sores

Ifo (water leaf) roots.
Grind roots.
Wash skin or sore constantly with infusion.

EGOPHIYO (INCANTATION)

In Urhobo medicine, especially in the treatment of social/preternatural and
supernatural diseases, the use of *Egophiyo* is prominent. Maclean opines that it
is in both traditional and orthodox systems of medicine that incantations are
employed. As she states it:

> For it is not only in the African situation that the use of medicine
> is accompanied by incantation. The instruction on how to use the
> medicine and the instruction itself on the bottle or envelope are all
> incantions [11]

The above statement underestimates the prominence and vitality of
egophiyo in Urhobo medicine. In the Urhobo context, the use of *egophiyo*
supersedes instructions. *Egophiyo* is the spoken word which has magical power
and when recited or chanted either on magical objects or alone, produces a
magical effect. *Egophiyo* is used in every aspect of human endeavour: economic,
political, social, and medicinal.

As I have mentioned above, both animate and inanimate objects or phenomena in the universe are imbued with life force which is the quintessence of the thing itself.[12] At the apex of the structural hierarchy is the Supreme Being whose spark gives the life force to other beings; followed by the divinities, spirits, ancestors, man; and at the lowest rug are the plants, animals, rocks, rivers, mountains and so on. Janheinz Jahn classifies these animate and inanimate objects into four categories, viz: *muntu* (man), *kintu* (thing), *hantu* (place and time) and kuntu (modality)[13]. *Muntu* consists of God, all human beings and the spirits. *Kintu* includes the animate and inanimate objects which are dormant and can be stimulated into action by a *muntu* by the use of the word. They are at the beck and call of man. Thus among all the created beings, it is only *ohwo* (man) who is created for his own sake while the other creatures are created for the sake of man. *Ohwo* is created as an end in himself. The absolute value man possesses is due to this; man is, therefore, willed for his own sake: he is the most perfect of all creatures and all the non-persons are willed for man.[14] The *kintu* forces are not self-willed because they lack intelligence which differentiates them from man. Once activated, the *kintu* can on their own influence other beings including man. Man differs from animals because of the word, and one man from another because each man uses the word relatively. Hence, the Urhobo say *Ota oye ohwo* (it is the word that differentiates one man from the other), *Egophiyo oye umwu* (the spoken word is the medicine; without it, there is no medicine).

In Urhobo medicine, the forces inherent in both animate and inanimate objects are activated by the use of *egophiyo* recited or chanted over them. In consonance with this concept, Janheinz Jahn writes:

> If there are no words, all forces would be frozen, there would be no procreation, no change, no life. Naming is an incantation, creative force. What we cannot conceive is unreal. It does not exist. But every human thought, once expressed becomes reality. The word holds the course of things in train and changes and transforms them.[15]

Man is imbued with intelligence and the power of the word which he exerts on the beings around him. He, therefore, employs them as a means to an end.[16]

The medicine man harnesses these qualities when he collects the *materia medica,* mentions what it is capable of performing, and what he intends the medicine to do. He also invokes *Oghene, edjo* and *esemo v 'iniemo* to bless and exercise their authorities over the medicine to ensure its efficacy. M. Iwu sees incantation and invocation as vehicles for raising the consciousness of the human mind especially the patient's.[17] Idowu on the other hand, has this to say about the attitude of the medicine man and his patient towards incantation and invocation of the spiritual beings.

> The point of the ritual is simply that unconsecrated medicine has no meaning for Africans. That is why divine and ancestral sanctions are

considered necessary before and during the preparation and application of medicine.[18]

The significance of the "word" in the Genesis creation story is summarized in M. Iwu's words:

> The word is before every other thing, in its fluid form it forms the material that fills the oceans and sacred rivers and also provides the soluble base for animal erythrocytes, including those of man. As fire, it erupts in volcanoes and gives teeth to lightening and thunders. The word in its simplest concept is a force effective and yet dormant until uttered.[19]

It was this dormant word that God uttered that created everything in the cosmos. He did not will it. The pre-existence of the word is well-articulated by the author of John's Gospel, when he says, "In the beginning was the Word, and the Word was with God..." (1: 1-3). The Biblical idea of the potency of the word has linkage with the Urhobo belief. In Urhobo medicine, the "word" activates or potentates the dormant life force in the *materia medica* and thus makes it efficacious. Janheinz Jahn summarised this concept thus:

> No medicine, "talisman", "magic horns", not even poisons are effective without the word. If they are not "conjured", they have no activity at all. Only the intelligence of the word frees these forces and makes them effective. All substances, animal, juice are only "vessel" of the word, of the Nommo.[20]

OBO, OBOEPHA, ORHERE (MEDICINE MAN, DIVINER AND PRIEST)

The paraxis of Urhobo traditional medicine is within the domain of three specialists - *Obo, Oboepha* and *Orhere* who include men and women. Mbiti[21] and Kokwora[22] observe that women often specialize in obstetrics, gynaecology, paediatrics, circumcision of girls and other general treatment while their male counterparts handle special cases like leprosy, abscess, gonorrhoea and so on. While Mbiti's and Kokwora's observation seems true, it does not apply to Madam Oti, who handles similar diseases.[23] In spite of these specialists, men of hidden supernatural power,[24] every household has the knowledge of some traditional medicine for the treatment of minor ailments such as headache, stomach troubles, fever, catarrh, cough, paediatrics, arthritis and other sicknesses believed to be caused naturally. It is in very serious and protracted sickness and disease that the attention and expert services of those men of hidden supernatural powers are needed.

Each of these specialists has his distinct role to perform in the Urhobo traditional medical system. The Urhobo perception of the aetiology of disease determines the role of each specialist. The *Obo*, basically heals through the utilization of medicine–roots, barks and leaves of plants, bones, birds, incantations and so on. The *Obo* possesses esoteric knowledge in the art of using flora and fauna materials including the supernatural forces to prevent and cure diseases. He also possesses good knowledge of medicine for the enhancement of life and of warding off malignant forces. Thus, to the African societies, the medicine men are the greatest gift and the most useful source of help..."He is accessible to everybody at all times"[25]. The Urhobo saying that *Omo r'obo ki ghwu ye ebe r'aghwa* (Before the child of a medicine man dies, there is no medicine or leaves left in the bush) attests to the wealth of knowledge acquired by Urhobo medical practitioners.

This esoteric knowledge is derived from training, revelation made by the ancestors, some from spirits while others may acquire it from their fathers or relatives who were *ebo* (plural of *obo*). Maclean[26] and Prince[27] indicate that native doctors come from families with long medical traditions, which families form the contemporary product of traditional Yoruba healing systems and the repositories of extensive medical lore. This statement is true of the Urhobo healers. For instance, Mume claims that he acquired his medical expertise from his grandmother's cousin, Ilarhe, who was a renowned traditional medicine man[28] while Madam Oti inherited it from her father.[29] Mr. E. Okpukoro explained how his father became a medicine man through his grandfather. He narrated how his dead grandfather showed his father a medicine with occultic power of removing thorns from the body without surgical operation in a dream.[30]

The *obo* with his knowledge of the various *materia medica*, the relationship between them, their combination and activation of their dormant forces through the utterance of the word, deserve to be designated a scientist. Margaret Field sees some relationship between traditional medicine and science. As she puts it: "We have seen that African medicine has, up to a point, a parallelism with science in that it is held that under certain defined conditions, certain defined results can be obtained irrespective of the person in charge of the operation".[31] Parrinder's statement is apposite when he says that the African medicine man:

> ...is a kind of scientist, in that he seeks to discover and use the laws of the universe, not only of an inanimate nature, but also of spiritual forces. He believes that there are powers that are hidden secret that can be tapped, not necessarily that he can force those powers to a different purpose, but there are laws which may be set in motion by the knowledgeable, as an electrician uses the forces of nature to light his house.[32]

It is the power of the *egophiyo* that sets the law of the universe in motion; and makes them acceptable to the supernatural beings. They, in turn, make the powers effective and render his medicine efficacious.[33]

Oboepha

The *oboepha* heals through the manipulation and interpretation of divination materials. The *oboepha*, a man with far-seeing eyes, is primarily concerned with the art of divination in an attempt to interpret the mysteries of life, to give guidance in daily affairs, to deliver the messages of the divinities, to uncover the past and pry into the future and to settle disputes.[34] Invariably, the *oboepha* is a diagnostician and at times combines the profession of *obo* while the *obo* is the physician/psychotherapist/spirit healer.[35]

The *obo* not only performs the role of a doctor and psychiatrist in the western societies, he is also an expert in spiritual forces by preparing protective charms against sorcerers, witches and evil forces and supplying medicines to attract good fortune – fertility, success in business and love affairs, good health. Distinctly, the *obo* performs four major roles – physician/psychotherapist, protector against forces of evil, healer of spiritual problems and provider of means of achieving one's aspirations.[36]

Orhere

The ministration of the *Orhere*, within the Urhobo medical system, is restricted to the performance of sacrifice which emanates from abominable offences committed against the supersensible forces and man. Ezeanya clearly brings out the role of the priest thus:

> A person who has committed an abominable act detestable to the divinities and man is really a sick person. Such acts like stealing particularly of commodities like yams, fowls and goats, murder, incest, adultery committed by a wife and such like offences are abominable acts and call for healing from the ministry of the priests.[37]

My interview with Mr. F. Ekama corroborates what Ezeanya has said. A man who bewitched and killed his wife and two daughters fell ill. It was a case of swollen body (oedema). He was taken to a hospital but could not avail himself of the treatment. A diviner was consulted to determine the cause of the illness. The diviner discovered it and the sick man was told to confess the sin he had committed and he did.

In the ritual that followed, the *Orhere* stated the offences before the ancestors, saying,

> *Umukoro fare ne oye hwe aye v'emete ive roye.*
> *Avware re ne ovwa, esemo na*
> *Vwe imwemu roye vwo rhovwo*
> *One oye bi rue otioye ofa-a.*[38]

Umukoro confessed that he killed his wife and two daughters. We are pleading that you, the ancestors forgive him his sins; that he would not do so again.

After the necessary sacrifice, the man became responsive to treatment and finally became well. This sacrifice was reluctantly performed because in most cases of this nature, the offender is left to suffer and die.

Human guilt accounts for one explanation of illness all over the world. "Guilt", according to Herjula, "is a state or position where a person is placed by his/her religion, culture or society after breaking a moral code, religious or social law or taboo."[39] It is religious, culture or society which defines guilt and it therefore belongs to cultural and social levels. This accounts for the relativity of taboos, as what is a taboo in one society may not be a taboo in another.

What is distinct in Urhobo medical practice is the absence of a divinity whose specific portfolio is medicine and divination. This contrasts the Yoruba *Orunmila* and *Osanyin* (divinities of divination and medicine) and the *Igbo Agwu* (divinity of diviners and medicine man).[40] While S.U Erivwo appreciates the use of leading questions as means of providing appropriate assessment of the client's situation by the *oboepha*, he never underplays the ability of some *eboepha* (plural) to tell their clients the purpose of their visit at first glance. As he argues it:

> For diviners have also been known to tell their clients the object of their mission at their first appearance, even before they had time to say anything; a phenomenon which would indicate that there is some element of telepathy in the process of divination. Because he uncovers the past, gives the cause of any calamity, and predicts the future by showing what powers in the other dimension have decreed, the diviner occupies an important position in the village and clan.[41]

However, Shorter views this power of telepathy as a means of creating confidence in the mind of the client but doubts the reliability of diviners.[42] Like in all professions, nobody doubts the presence of charlatans, but the truth is that the majority of the diviners in Urhoboland are reliable.

The Urhobo perception of disease is holistic and the healing is multi-dimensional and integrative. The Urhobo medical practitioners hardly make any clear distinction between the different levels in which they operate — physical, emotional, psychic, social and religious. They can operate on all these levels at once. This is considered the greatest benefit of traditional medical system. These medical specialists were the focal point of attack and campaign of vilification by the missionaries. They viewed them as the propagators of superstition and magic. They were thus designated sorcerers, magicians and witch-doctors. But today, the missionary attack and campaign have been proved to be due to total ignorance arising from their inability to comprehend thoroughly what traditional medicine means to the people.

The pathological state used to be the focus of orthodox medicine and the state of the mind was thought not to affect the well-being of the body. But today, orthodox medicine acknowledges the influence of the mind and the social environment on the healing pattern of patients. It now employs psychological and spiritual treatment in its healing process. Maclean asserts that whereas it is only relatively recently that western medicine has come to acknowledge the importance of psychosomatic factors in illness, this has for long permeated African medicine.[43] It is apparent that the hubris of science is thinning out gradually and thus the main point of difference between the Urhobo and western scientific cosmologies. And Horton succinctly points out that:

> Modern medicine man, though long blinded to such things by the fantastic success of the germ theory of disease, are once more beginning to toy with the idea that disturbances in a person's social life can in fact contribute to a whole series of sickness, ranging from those commonly thought of as mental to many more thought of as bodily. In making this rediscovery, however, the medical men have tended to associate it with the so-called pressures of modern living.[44]

To cater for sickness arising from psychosomatic factors, many chaplaincy and counselling centres have been built into orthodox medicine centres.

In Christianity, healing is believed to proceed from God. In the Apocrypha, Ecclesiasticus Chapter 38 verses 1-15 is the famous passage about the physician:

> Honour the physician with the honour due to him...for the Lord created him; for healing comes from the Most High... the Lord created medicines from the earth, and a sensible man will not despise them. He gave skill to men that they might be glorified in his marvellous works... There is a time when success leaps in the hand of the physicians, for they too will pray to the Lord that he should grant them success in diagnosis and in healing, for the sake of preserving life...[45]

This Old Testament concept of healing sees sickness as caused by sin and the need to return to God. The first thing to do is to turn to God in repentance who heals through the physician. This is similar to what operates in the Urhobo medical practice.

The Ministry of Jesus underscored the significance of life. Healing, as means of preserving, enhancing and controlling of diseases which destabilize it, formed its central part. Goodchild remarks that one fifth of the gospel consists of accounts of physical and mental healing.[46] Like every other healing practice, faith is the bedrock for the acceptance and appropriation of the power of Jesus. In Paul's ministry to the gentiles, healing was also performed. It was one of the reasons why Paul had to choose Luke, a physician to take care of his personal health problems.

The church today is fully committed to healing ministry. The independent churches are bestriding the areas of continuity between Urhobo and Christian religions. Some independent churches emphasize the power of prayer and ritual to the total exclusion of the use of medicine. Others accept the use of tablets for treatment of physical/natural diseases while emphasizing that psychosomatic diseases require rituals, fasting, prayers and the patient needs cleansing from sins. Their explanation of causality is based mainly on the machination of spirits which are present in the universe especially witchcraft and sorcery. Iwuagwu attributes the heavy leaning on scientific medicine to total ignorance of the aetiology of diseases and sickness. As he puts it:

> As this lip service given to it (healing ministry) is due to the fact that we rely on scientific medication for almost every illness. We ignore the fact that some illnesses do not respond to scientific medicine. Illnesses that are psychological or spiritual, defy ordinary diagnosis. Such illnesses can rather be diagnosed through psychological or spiritual methods.[47]

He, therefore, advises that church healing ministry should reactivate the whole man through the reciting or chanting of incantation, that is prayers. Hence he observes that:

> The Church healing ministry must reactivate the whole man. Healing of the body or of the mind in order to give health to an individual. If the activation is medical, it operates from the body, if psychological, healing may be achieved by the suggestion or by stimulating the soul or by calming the emotional centre of the sick. If spiritual, the reactivation of the body or the mind is brought about by an external spiritual power, who by Christian identification is God.[48]

The different aspects of man which, Iwuagwu argues, need cure in order to bring about the wholeness of man have long been the focus of Urhobo medicine. This is mainly responsible for why many scholars have paid tribute to traditional medical practice. They view it as a potential and fertile ground from which orthodox medical practice can cultivate and yield a bumper harvest.[49] As Una Maclean rightly puts it:

> To direct attention in the study of African medicine, solely upon the pharmacologically active component of herbal medicine is not to sift what is scientifically valuable from the dross of irrelevance. The enduring value of African medicine lies not in its materials but in the methods and concept which underlie them and its continuity power is a tribute to the practitioners of this ancient art.[50]

This ancient art of the Urhobo can only be understood through a thorough understanding of the Urhobo cosmology.

From the above analysis, it is tacit that Urhobo medicine and its practitioners were misunderstood and misinterpreted by the westerners. This error of judgement was consequent on the fact that the early missionaries, anthropologists and ethnographers emerged from a scientific cosmology, **which** is at variance with the Urhobo cosmology that is essentially religious. This inability to understand the traditional cosmology afforded the use of perjorative terms such as superstitions, juju, fetish, etc. to describe Urhobo medicine. The practitioners of traditional medicine were dubbed witch–doctors/hunters, magicians, sorcerers, and their clients regarded as ignorant. For the most part, their medicines were regarded as inefficacious. This is the point which Ezeabisili has against the foreign writers and describes their theses as propaganda.[51] It is to avoid misinterpretation and misunderstanding in the study of traditional medicine that Una Maclean warns that:

> African medicine can only be properly understood in its complete cultural context since the way in which people respond to illness or misfortune in any culture is inevitably related to the whole religious and philosophical framework in which existence is perceived.[52]

The study of medicinal plants currently in vogue has revealed that plants used by the traditional medical practitioners contain active principles which effect the cure of the disease. Thus traditional medicines have been proved to be efficacious. The image of traditional medicine practitioners and their clients as described by Professor Iwu above has been laid to rest.

The use of *egophiyo* (incantation) in Urhobo medicine was also assaulted by the western writers. It has been pointed out that *egophiyo* has universal usage even in orthodox medicine and in the Christian healing ministry especially in their prayers. While Maclean relates the use of incantations to instructions and prescriptions in orthodox medicine, in traditional medicine and Christian healing ministry, their usage comprehend more than that. Incantations in the latter two healing processes set the dormant forces in the *kintu* (animal, trees, rocks, etc) in motion and effectuate the desired goal. *Egophiyo* in this respect, especially in the traditional context, relates to all aspects of life and can even ward off the evil forces that may cause illness.

There is much linkage between traditional medicine and the Christian healing ministry. As I have mentioned above, the use of *egophiyo* is prominent in both. Both relate causal explanation of disease to spiritual, physical, and emotional factors arising from breakdown in interpersonal relationship. Orthodox and traditional medical practitioners undergo a period of apprenticeship, in order to acquire the requisite knowledge and techniques for their professions. In both, minor ailments are attended to within the family, but in the case of protracted ones, the expert services of the practitioners are sought.

The differences and linkages noted above emanated from differences in cultural backgrounds in which they are operational. Whereas the western scientific cosmology dictates scientific modes, the western writers failed to relate traditional medicine to traditional cosmology, the understanding of which would have been the open sesame to traditional medicine. To appreciate Urhobo traditional medicine therefore, requires a thorough knowledge of the Urhobo cosmology.

RITUAL AND EFFICACY IN URHOBO MEDICINE

The Urhobo, like all other peoples in the world over, have always had a well-developed and effective medical system. The Urhobo call medicine *umu, umwu* or *uhuvwu*, depending on dialect differentiation. It is this medical system which sustained and still sustains the Urhobo. It is estimated that about 90% of the rural population of many developing countries derive their health care from traditional medicine.[53] That notwithstanding, we find that at times some of these people opt for western medical care, where traditional medicine fails to meet their expectation.

As noted already above, traditional medicine deals with the totality of the patient's socio-cultural, spiritual and psychological framework. In treating the patient, the healers employ methods of restoring the total personality by allaying his fears, anxiety, stress and strain. Margaret Mead describes the personal interest of the healer in the patient and how important he tries to create an atmosphere of confidence and trust to allay the anxiety felt by the patient and his friends. The healer does not only speak to the patient and relatives in the language they understand but also applies concepts familiar to them.[54] This indicates the involvement of many rituals in the treatment modalities of Urhobo healer. Therapy through rituals (charm medicine) has been viewed with much scepticism by the westerners, some Nigerian elites and orthodox Christians because it is at variance with Aristotle's syllogism and reason models.[55] However, Nze has vouched for the reliability of charm medicine:

> If it is difficult to deny the evidence that human mind can make connection with space, time and matter in ways which have nothing to do with the ordinary sense, and if science, for example, physics itself is much more magical and bizarre and yet is recognized and accepted, then charm medicine (ritual therapy) should be granted favourable audience.[56]

The efficacy of African medicine has been proved. As early as 1920, Father Julian Gorju had attested to this by saying that traditional healers did not have the slightest idea about matter of dosages but that their remedies were astonishingly efficacious.[57] Dr. S. Akinnulli's remark also demonstrates the efficacy of the African medicine. As he puts it:

> The main objectives in any art of healing is the ultimate achievement of a lasting cure. In fact, there have been many cases where orthodox medicine failed and the traditional medicine proved useful in the treatment of chronic diseases.[58]

A. E. Ohiaeri is more specific in reporting the efficacy of Nsukka snake bite remedy.

> So, far, we have treated in the University Medical Centre, six victims of the bite from this dangerous snake (Carpet viper, Nsukka's most dangerous snake). In all the six cases, the cure was rapid and

completely effective. All the patients described the relief from the pain as taking approximately seven minutes after the administration of the remedy which is taken orally. No relapse occurred.[59]

M. Gelfand also reported of a medicine woman who effectively treated cases of asthma with a stramonium leaf and yet she lived in a very remote village.[60] The efficacy of traditional medicine has been widely acclaimed by Professor Lambo, Dr. Folayele Awosika, a specialist in clinical pharmacy and herbal medicine, Abimbola Sodipe, National President of the Nigerian Union of Medical Herbal Practitioners,[61] Raymond Prince, Pa Jimoh Esukoya, T. Hockmayer, Dopamu,[62] among others. This also is the attestation of my interviewees. The efficacy of ritual therapy is tied to the use of words of intention. Man as a *homo loquens* and *homo volens* (talking and willing being) can through the use of the word activate the dormant forces inherent in both animate and inanimate objects and harness them for man's weal or woe.[63]

With the above remarks and observations, the efficacy of traditional medicine including ritual therapy is indubitable. In its treatment of diseases, everyone sees the response of the patient to the treatment. This forms the basis for judging the efficacy or otherwise of traditional medicine.[64]

Ritual

V.W. Turner defines ritual as "prescribed formal behaviour for occasions not given over to technological routine having reference to beliefs in mystical beings or power."[65] Turner's definition is vitiated because he forgets that ritual is universal since man by nature is a ritual being. He had defined ritual from the perspective of the less developed cultures. Even in the orthodox medical system which is highly technological, there are rituals to be performed or observed before a surgical operation. Thus a devout Christian surgeon might say his prayers quietly or even make the sign of the cross before commencing a surgical operation. Some of the rituals in traditional healing were of necessity directed to the same goal; to invoke the name of God, divinities and ancestors to make effective and curative the treatment to be given.

Shorter's definition indicates the universality of ritual. He defines ritual as "literary or verbal symbols accompanied with symbolic action. Human beings everywhere fundamentally try to act out their expectations or experiences through symbolic action".[66] Ritual is a nexus between verbal symbols and man's daily activities and at the same time participates in their nature. Ritual gives purpose to man's activities and humanizes them. Through rituals, man is capable of reinserting himself into reality and ritual assists him to restore order to society. Hence, Monica Wilson sees rituals as "the key to an understanding of the essential constitution of human society."[67] Ritual may also be defined as a specific, observable kind of behaviour based on established or traditional rules.[68] Ritual is also capable of giving meaning to the experiences of mankind that otherwise could be contradictory. The resolution of this contradiction is achieved through adequate reference to the transcendental otherness. Ritual aids the revelation of the social values of the religious community and communicate same to the participants. They indicate the structure of a community, its ontological hierarchy, the rights and obligations of the members and their relationship including transcendental realities.[69] It is in consonance with the functions of rituals that Zuesse observes: "African spirituality, above and beyond the specific focus of particular ritual actions, is always a piety directed towards the sanctity of the universe as a whole."[70]

Rituals are classed into two categories, viz, religious and secular. Religious rituals are those which appeal to spiritual being; secular rituals, on the other hand, are those which make no appeal to spiritual beings. This classificatory model is fluid since many rituals participate in elements from both the secular and religious. The occurrence of any calamity or affliction in a social group warrants taking measures to restore the status *quo ante*. In such a case, recourse is had to a diviner to ferret the causes and prescribe appropriate rituals to be performed.

Efficacy

Webster's Third New International Dictionary defines efficacy as "the power to produce an effect". That efficacy is synonymous with effectiveness. In any medical system, especially traditional medicine, the efficacy of a therapy is the result of the combination of two powers, viz; the power of the herbs (90% of all remedies)[71] and the power of the medicine man. The double power derives from rituals relating to the production and preservation of the medicine. These rituals include the collection of the *materia medica* at specific times, at times accompanied with liquor or liquid, the preparation of the remedy under specific conditions and its preservation in special area. Sometimes the ritual involves the hand to be used in lifting the medicine to the mouth, as well as the manner and number of times the remedy must be taken. However, it is not all therapies that involve serious rituals. The adoption of ritual in the Urhobo medical system is consequent on the nexus between magic, medicine and religion.

RITUAL AS AN INTRINSIC PART OF URHOBO MEDICINE

Ritual as an intrinsic part of Urhobo medicine is effective in the treatment of diseases that are within the spiritual, psychosocial and moral levels. For instance, a man had a problem in getting a wife. All his advances to prospective partners were rebuffed. He was, however, told by a medicine man to perform some rituals that his problem would be solved if somebody was responsible. The traditional doctor told him to get a centipede, go to an intersection and whirl the centipede round his head seven times while saying:

Obo ri kpokpo vwe eje
Ro nerhe vwe je aye evwo na
Erhivwi na sie aye eje no nure
Kirobo r'ohwo sa rie erhivwi na
Eriyi ohwo ovuovo se ru vwe emu vuovo-o
Obo ri mi she erhivwi na etine none na
Eriyi obo re soro eje ro nerhe vwe
Je aye evwo na eje eji she aye jtine none na.[72]

Everything that is responsible for my inability to get a wife.
The centipede has cleansed them all.
As a centipede is inedible so also I have become impregnable.
As I have buried the centipede here today so also have
I buried all the problems associated with my inability to get a wife.

At the seventh time, he should bury the centipede at the intersection. After this ritual, he should take granulated sugar, soap and sponge to a stream to bathe. While bathing he should say:

Kemu kemu ro soro nerhe vwe je aye evwo
ahworhere kofia none ki none yara eyere me ve
ihwo efa ko dia miemie kiro oyubu

Everything associated with my inability to get a wife is cleansed today,
As from today, my relationships with other people should be as sweet as sugar.

He should sponge himself from head to toe while repeating the *egophiyo* (words of intention).

The gentleman went, performed the ritual and today he is happily married with children. This same ritual was also performed by an applicant who was unsuccessful in a number of interviews he attended. He also became successful in the first interview after he had performed the ritual.[73]

The Urhobo's belief that someone could make life miserable for others is well illustrated in the two examples above. No doubt, these two gentlemen were touched with an anti-social medicine which the Urhobo call *utuoma* (medicine for hatred) so that anybody who had close relationship with them might hate them, for no just cause.

The second illustration is that of a son who became sick. All effective medicines were applied but the sickness became more serious. He was taken to a modern hospital where the doctors told his relatives that the sickness was not a hospital case; that he should be sent for traditional treatment. The father became so worried that he went to consult *oboepha* (diviner) who told him that the son had committed a sin against the ancestors; that he would not survive the sickness if he failed to confess it. The father went home and convinced the son to confess the sin he had committed. After much persuasion, the son confessed that he had had sexual intercourse with his father's wife and stolen the father's money.

The elders of the family met, fined the son a goat, seven tubers of yam and a substantial sum of money. In the ritual that follows, the *paterfamilas*, (the head of the extended family) recounted the confessions of the son to the ancestors as follows:

> *Odemero fare ne oyechi igho re'ose roye re duvwi iyori ho*
> *Oje fa ne oye ji due aye r'ose roye*
> *Avware kokori none re vwo reovwa*
> *Ese ve ini r'avware ne wa vwe imwemu*
> *R'Odemero ruru vwo rhovwo fikiridie omotete orue.*[74]

Odemero has confessed that he stole his father's money for which he appealed to you to intervene. Odemero also confessed that he had sexual dealings with his father's wife (the name of wife is always mentioned). We, the elders of the family have gathered today to plead with you, our fathers and mothers to forgive the sins Odemero has committed, because Odemero is senseless.

It was after the sacrifice that further medication proved efficacious and the son later became well.

During my research work in 1986, I was informed about how a breakdown in relationship between son's wife and her mother-in-law led to the former's delayed labour. The diviner who was consulted told the woman's relatives that she had insulted her mother-in-law and that the unborn baby was insisting that its mother should settle with its grandmother by buying a wrapper for her. Immediately, the wrapper was given to the mother-in-law and she prayed for her safe delivery, the woman's sister gave a birth to a bouncing baby boy.[75]

I have discussed elsewhere how a father who had incest with his daughter when they travelled overseas was taken ill. He was taken to hospitals and traditional doctors for treatment but all were to no avail. People saw in dreams the ugly relationship he had with his daughter and told him to confess but he never did. In the final analysis, the man died and until 1985 when I carried out the research, the daughter had not given birth to any child.[76] This important man died because the rituals intrinsic to Urhobo medicine and which could have rendered other treatment efficacious were not performed because he failed to confess his sin in good time.

Examples of how rituals aid the efficacy of Urhobo medicine could be multiplied. It is these examples of preternatural treatment that are often called magic by the westerners. To them, they are representative examples of irrationality and malpractice, a mixture of superstition and deliberate deception and ignorance.[77] E.B. Tylor caricatured them as a monstrous farrago containing no truth or value whatsoever.[78] The westerners described this type of medicine and treatment in these derogatory terms because they were ignorant and would not understand their working and efficacy. However, Shorter had warned against this sceptical attitude found among foreigners and social scientists, who by their training and professions are sceptical, advising that they also should preserve an open mind and be ready to admit irrefutable evidence that magic really works; and that events anticipated in symbolic rite really occur.[79]

RITUAL AS AN EXTRINSIC PART OF URHOBO MEDICINE

I have mentioned above that the treatment of natural diseases, does not involve many rituals except the peripheral. These rituals are the characteristics of herbalists and medical doctors. Peripheral rituals are meant to reinforce the remedy in the treatment process. For instance, fracture is a naturally caused disease. In my interview with a traditional orthopaedic doctor, he indicated that there was no ritual associated with his treatment.[80] However, from his description of the process, I discovered that the treatment is completely devoid of ritual. For instance, the breaking of hen's leg and using medicine to tie it has nothing to do with the treatment of the fracture; rather it makes the patient well disposed to the treatment.

Let us illustrate. In the preparation of a certain remedy for gonorrhoea, a broom stick must be tied on the neck of a bottle while it is in the centre of a circle drawn with a kaolin (native chalk). Seven spices (*Urierie*) and the bark of the tree procured fresh from the bush are put into the bottle before *ogogoro* or any hot drink is poured on the mixture. This medicine was later prepared by another friend without observing the ritual (tying a broom stick on the neck of the bottle, putting the bottle in the centre of a circle drawn with native chalk, and without being specific about the number "seven" of *urierie* (spices)) and yet it worked.[81]

The analysis of the ritual demonstrates that the remedy treats both natural and preternatural gonorrhoea. The broom stick sweeps out all malignant forces while the circle excludes all mystical evil forces and renders the environment sacrosanct. Having excluded all mystical evil forces, the efficacy of the herbal preparation is ensured. The preparation of the medicine without the ritual and its efficacy indicate that the man's gonorrhoea was natural. It also shows the difference between a professional and amateur healer. As Mbiti rightly points out:

> The medicine man offers a prayer as he treats the sick, indicating that God is ultimately the healer. It is a common belief among many traditional medicinemen that they do not wield final power for healing the sick and only use the powers, skills, knowledge, and medicines given to them by God. Some of them are known to include prayer as part of their medical practice; and in addition, some make offering and sacrifice, or perform other religious rituals, in connection with their work.[82]

This attitude of dependence of the finite and contingent being on the infinite and absolute Being is not only peculiar to the Urhobo traditional medical practitioners but to all *homo sapiens* including the agnostics. Thus orthodox doctors and other medical personnel pray so that God might attend their treatment with success because He is the determiner of all destinies. This attitude is also exhibited in all aspects of life.

Another similar example was that given by Venerable Archdeacon N. A. Enuku, the Bishop of Warri Diocese (1992). His mother has medicine for treating swollen legs (oedema). However, Bishop Enuku later prepared it for a person but this time with fire ashes because native chalk was not available and yet it was efficacious.[83]

A third illustration was when my mother showed me a very effective medicine for treating bones and nerves. It is a simple medicine but at the end of it all, she added that if l wanted to conceal it from other persons that l could pluck other leaves and add to it or perform any other ritual.[84]

The examples here indicate that remedies for treating natural/physical diseases contain active principles which cure such diseases. For instance, without the rituals in the above treatment of natural diseases, the remedies will also be effective. As it has been argued above, the Urhobo believe that natural diseases are fertile ground for the agents of preternatural diseases to operate. The involvement of rituals in some of the examples above is therefore an attempt by the healer to approach the treatment from different dimensions based on the Urhobo perception of diseases. Rituals, which are inherent or inevitably present in such treatments, have marked out Urhobo medicine as a distinct therapeutic system. Such rituals cannot be disassociated from the Urhobo therapeutic system; otherwise the whole system crumbles; because therapy through rituals— psychosocial level—is built on group symbols and the people's belief system. Hence Iwu remarks that healing is part of African religion, that there is a peculiar unity of religion and life that is essentially African; and that healing is concerned with the restoration or preservation of human vitality, wholeness and continuity.[85] Iwu's remark points out the significance of ritual in Urhobo African medical systems.

REASONS FOR RITUALS IN URHOBO MEDICINE

The point has been made that the use of rituals is universal and that they function in order to serve some purposes. The role of ritual discussed below is not exclusively related to Urhobo medicine but to all medical systems.

Ritual serves as a point of contact with the supernatural beings that promote the healing process. During the preparation and administration remedy, the Urhobo healer summons *Oghene, edjo and esemo v'iniemo* to bless and make the medicine efficacious. The ancestors were those who first used the medicine and later passed it to their progeny. Now possessing some extraneous power than ordinary mortals, the ancestors could make the treatment effective and also assist in the removal of all evil forces that might impede its efficiency.

Ritual promotes psychological conditioning which facilitates acceptance of the healing capacity of the treatment. Studies have revealed that the social and the psychological conditions surrounding a patient are so momentous that they can be responsible for a patient's full recovery or he may relapse and remain in an unhealthy state. It can, therefore, be argued that the traditional healers realized earlier than their western counterparts that psychotherapy is an essential and dynamic basis for effective system of treatment. Ritual not only enables us to assess the relationship between the medicine man and patient but also enables the medicine man to investigate the cultural, social, intellectual milieu and the background of the patient. Well armed with evidence arising therefrom, the Urhobo healers can evaluate and interpret the cause of the diseases and give necessary assistance. Dopamu equals this attitude to medical psychology.[86]

Ritual functions in order to establish a unity of forces, a single purpose of minds of the traditional doctor and patient towards one focus, that is, the achievement of success in the healing process. Ritual aids in convincing the healer and patient that the healer is capable of handling his case. Thus faith is an indispensable tool in all medical systems.

Ritual helps to establish contact with the patient's mind by tapping his belief system and cultural endowments. To the Urhobo man, an unconsecrated medicine is thought inefficacious since the three dimensions of cause of diseases are always present in his mind. Ritual, therefore, assists in disposing the mind of the patient towards the treatment.

Apart from these latent or ideational functions of ritual, ritual is efficacious in the Urhobo medical system in actually securing successful healing. This function of ritual is noteworthy in supernaturally and psychosocially caused diseases and their treatments.

COMPARATIVE ANALYSIS OF THE EFFICACIOUS USE OF RITUAL IN URHOBO AND WESTERN MEDICAL SYSTEMS

We have emphasized the role of ritual in creating confidence and consequently faith in both the healer and the patient as a *sine qua non* in all medical systems. The Urhobo cosmology is religious and in all religions, man realizes his limitations and to succeed in life, he must be in good relationship with the supersensible realities. It is for this reason, the Urhobo man tries to invoke the Supreme Being, divinities and ancestors in whatever he does. Thus, in Urhobo medical system, the use of rituals is predominant.

In the preparation and administration of medicament, the Supreme Being whom the healer believes imbues the *materia medica* with the active principles must be summoned. The divinities who must have revealed the medicine to the healer in a dream or vision must be called upon to participate in the treatment process. The ancestors who had practised the medicine and later on passed the process to the healer are not left out. Secondly, the Urhobo believe that some external agents like witches, sorcerers, ancestors, and divinities cause diseases. If the treatment is to be effective, the healer believes, these agents must be appeased through sacrifice and other related rituals. All these rituals are performed so as to create confidence and faith not only in himself but also in the patient. Thus sacrifices, incantations and prayers are commonly used in Urhobo medicine.

In the healing ministry of the believers, rituals and the use of *egophiyo* (incantation) abound. Prayers are said in order to cast away evil forces from the environment, patients are told to believe that Jesus can heal them of all their infirmities before ritual cleansing with water or olive oil.

In the western medical system, with its emphasis on empirical verification of evidence guided by a body of explicit acceptance/rejection criteria, the use of ritual is attenuated. However, before any surgical operation, a Christian Surgeon might say his prayers and assure the patient of a successful operation. The patient is psychologically worked up to have confidence in the medicines. There are cases of some patients with serious ailment who were given placebo treatment and became well. Counselling units are now built in orthodox hospitals.

In the mission hospitals, chaplaincy has been attached to them to effectively work up the patients psychologically by allaying their fears and to mitigate their perception of aetiology of disease that Jesus can heal it all. In the Baptist Hospital, Eku (the only mission hospital in Urhoboland), short prayers and sermon are usually given on clinic days. The patients are told that the medicines they have been given are not different from others they have been taking before. But that they should believe that Jesus can heal them. It must be emphasized that the function of all these rituals, whether in Urhobo or in Western medical system, is to create faith and confidence in both the healer and the patient.[87]

CONCLUSION

Urhobo medicine is practised in a dynamic culture which is constantly in flux; if traditional medicine is to be developed to an international level of acceptance, what will be the prospect of the rituals? Nowadays, both the federal and state governments and private entrepreneurs are being urged to invest in traditional medicine because of the immense advantages that will accrue not only to them but also to the generality of the Nigerian populace. For instance, it is being argued that such investments will assist in providing regular supply of drugs, thereby solving the problem of shortage of drugs and equipment plaguing our medical centres. It will also serve as a foreign reserve earner to the country and reduce the amount of money expended on the importation of drugs. Awosika also added his lonely voice by calling on the governments to do something concrete about the development of traditional medicine: "Despite the huge sums of money spent on importing drugs and equipment, our medical centres still lack essential drugs and equipment. And this is particularly why government should pay attention to traditional medicine and its practitioners".[88]

Some advancement is, however, being made by the traditional medicine practitioners to make their medicines into capsules and cough syrup for both children and adults. In using these capsules, no serious ritual is performed unlike when the patient had approached the healer himself. Here again, S. N. Enunuaye argued that the *egophiyo* (incantation) and other necessary rituals had been communicated into the capsules and cough syrups by the traditional practitioner and that such medicines could be effective.[89] The import of Mr. Enunuaye's argument is that the use of ritual in Urhobo medicine is scientific even where it is extrinsic to treatment, since it is useful in the culture in which it is applied.

Acupuncture, the Chinese traditional medical system, is today enjoying international recognition. The Chinese government and people encouraged and developed it. By gaining international acceptance, the system, no doubt, must have divested itself of the early trappings (rituals) which hitherto trammelled it within the Chinese cultural milieu. Today, literate Christians, Moslems and agnostics patronize it. Funny enough, however, most Christians, elites and agnostics condemn traditional medicine as superstitious, mostly because of the many rituals it entails. Since culture with all its elements (including its medical system) is dynamic, traditional medicine and its practitioners should be prepared to align themselves to the wind of change. In this way, many of the irrelevant rituals which are believed to be trade gimmicks of the professional healers will either be obliterated or mitigated. The Urhobo (Africans) have to re-educate themselves that the rituals are efficacious to Urhobo (African) medicine. Consequently, Urhobo (African) traditional medicine will emerge as internationally accepted therapeutic system. Urhobo (Africans) shall have then contributed its quota to medicine.

The list of the mystical medicine below may be designated magic since they do not cure any specific disease. But inasmuch as they assist man in enhancing his life and to realize his life aspirations, in the Urhobo context, they are called *umwu/uhuvwu* (medicine). It is for this reason that they have been so designated. We have decided to substitute the term *mystical medicine* for *magical medicine* because *materia medica* with active principles are used. We note that the designation "magical" is repudiated because the European definition and use of *magic* refer to means of conjuring.

Mystical Medicine for	Materia Medica	Preparation	Administration
Udidi (awe) also prevention against witchcraft.	*Uloho* (Iroko tree/ seven young leaves, one seed of alligator pepper, a bucket of water and a stick with fire.	Put all items inside bucket of water and squeeze leaves, put stick with fire inside the bucket of water. Throw the stick to your front and if the part with fire faces the person, it is a sign that the medicine will not be effective. Pick stick again and throw it until the part with fire points outside.	Use concoction to bathe while saying the following incantation *"Odidi ro obi eje mue obi i. Ame boroboro oye furhie erhare."* (Nobody can hold cobra because of its awe, even if water is insipid, it quenches fire).
Useki (Medicine for attracting customers).	*Iku* (cray-fish), seven *irhibo vwievwie,* seven small pepper and water.	Squeeze all items in water while saying this incantation: *"Eji ineki me bu none na kere iku kugbe irhibo vwievwie."*	Bathe with water before going for sales. While saying: " *Eji ineki me bu none na kere iku kugbe irhibo vwievwie."* (Let my customers be as many as crayfish and small pepper).
Prevention against enemies, attack (cutlass -proof).	*Arhua* (leaves) 7 alligator pepper seeds Praying *metisi* egg bag.	Chew items together	Swallow everything

Mystical Medicine for	Materia Medica	Preparation	Administration
Protection against witchcraft and other enemies.	*Obuko iyeke, ivwrevwre, ikweku re aderha,* native cola nut (3 lobes), *Ogogoro* and breakable pot, water.	Put all items in the pot and add water and mix all together while saying these incantations: *"Obuko iyeke da mo. Ivwrevwre vwe esiri-i. Ohwo ro tue ohwo odi te aderha ko whre. Oghene ovwata na mo wo ri gwedjo nana."*	After the preparation and the incantation, wash with the decoction while reciting the incantation and invocation of God at a cross road.
Protection against sorcerers, witchcraft and attack of enemies.	Seven leaves of *Akalamudo* (not allowed to fall to the ground while collecting them), water collected from a trunk of a tree (any stagnant water) a leaf that falls and decomposed in water, any seven leaves from a live tree, one seed of alligator pepper and a native pot.	Put all items in the pot one after the other while saying this incantation: *"Akalamudo waruyovwi ko owhee, obe ro she phiho ame ro dje-a etiye ogbo phiho, ihwo ive ghara ibe re rhire-e Ogbene ovwata na kugbe esemo warhe ri gwedjo nana."*	The pot including the items should be carried to the cross road. Bathe with water while reciting the incantation. *Akalamudo* does not shave hair for flood, a leaf that falls inside a stagnant water usually decomposes in it. Two people do not share one alligator pepper, God of justice and the ancestors come and judge this case. After bathing, carry pot and whirl it round head and leave it in the midair to fall and break. Move away immediately without looking back.

Mystical Medicine for	Materia Medica	Preparation	Administration
Cooling down some one's temper or to judge a case in one's favour.	One yam, 2 padlocks, *owhre* (fish) tread, kola nut, *orhe* (native chalk), the leaves in which a rabbit sleeps, the first leaf out of the seven usually found under the head of puff adder *(ovwe)*, (snake).	Grind items together and rub keys with medicine. The person then prays for what he wishes to happen. The yam and the head of the *owhre* (fish) are cooked together while saying *owhre* has no mouth to born. Collect any water from yam in a bottle.	Tie all items together. Use yam water to serve the medicine while reciting incantation before going to the court, or meeting the man who is annoyed with you.
Cutlassproof for 24 hours *erhenede Etuwevwi* (prevention against motor accident). Protection against armed robbers.	*Enyaubaka,* (Grasshopper's egg sack), seven seeds of alligator, caterpillar cocoon, black tread, *isoro nogbo* (catsheat) *Akpobrisi,* one fly).	Grind together, tie all items together. Recite this incantation: *"a mrasa mre ohori rohe uwevwi roye-e"* Nobody can see caterpillar in its cocoon.	Say this incantation: "I, *Ukpede esivwe, Opia rohwo sa ro vwe none-e."* It is only today. Nobody's cutlass can cut me, spray and hide item in your pocket.
Vomiting of poison.	*Ikpamuku* (flower). (African Marigold), palm kernels (7) and alligator pepper (7 seeds).	Chew items together.	Swallow chewed items.

Mystical Medicine for	Materia Medica	Preparation	Administration
Securing a job.	*Umako* leaves (pepper fruit), palm kernel (twin type),-a penny salt, candle (7) and a basin.	Break kernel until twin type is got. Take that that falls to the right. Wash leaves in a basin. Chew the kernel and spray the basin while saying: *"Uwheriaka nerhe emu miemie"* (7 times). This means salt sweetens food.	Bathe with infusion at the backyard while saying: *Uwheriaka nerhe emu miemie* ''(7 times). Salt sweetens food. Light one candle at night and sleep alone till dawn for seven days.
Okpo Cutlass-proof.	*Ikpamaku* (flowers) (African Marigold), alligator pepper (7).	Chew all items	Swallow chewed items
Okpo Cutlass-proof.	*Ishasha* (leaves). (7) (Black pepper), alligator pepper (7 seeds), one native egg.	Wash leaves and boil egg.	Chew leaves, alligator pepper and egg. **Taboo:** Do not eat egg with another person. Avoid eating raw palm nut. Avoid daytime sexual intercourse.
Court case and to face a panel.	*Egbri* (lawn grass), the forehead of a native cow (*erhue*)	Uproot it with right foot, add the hairs and make a knot while saying: *"Arha rhara ana erhue"* (7x). It is the forehead of the native cow one only looks at, you cannot do anything. to it.	Put tied knot in your pocket and proceed to court or to face the panel. **Taboo:** Do not greet anybody on the way until you are called in the court or by the panel. You should also say the incantations in your mind.

Mystical Medicine for	Materia Medica	Preparation	Administration
Court Case.	*ebe eti* (7 times), *evwererha* (three lobed kolanut), alligator pepper (7 seeds) and one needle.	Hold seven leaves together and pin it to a wall. Break kolanut, chew each lobe and add alligator pepper and chew all items together.	Spray chewed items on pinned leaves on the wall and go to the court.
Cure of poison or unidentified sickness or disease.	*Obuko iyeke,* (leaves) *Oluku* or *egberebo* root, roots of water lettuce, *ofuako, Ubophe* (flower and scraping), strong native salt. **Reaction:** vomiting	Grind all items together including strong native salt, Put inside bottle, add water or *ogogoro.* Shake bottle Before drinking, running stomach should not be feared, urine also turns yellow.	Drink twice a day, i.e morning and before bed. **Reaction:** vomiting, or excessive excreting.

Names of some Medicinal Plants in Urhobo Cultural Areas

North Eastern Formerly Ethiope Local Govt. Area.	North-Western Okpe Uvwie	Southern Formerly Ugheli Local Govt. Area	South-Eastern, Orogun
Achavwe	Achavwe	Achavwe	Achavwe
Ayovwe	Ayovwe	Ayovwe	Ayovwe
Ehirhe	Ewho	Ehirhe, ewho	Ewho
Eke	Eke	Eke	Eke
Egberebo	Egberebo	Egberebo	Egberebo
Eshasha	Erharha	Eshasha	Ozeze
Eran	Eberierhiarhian	Eran	Ororotan
Erevwereba	Imeren	Erevwereba	Ilasa
Erhie	Erhie	Erhie	Erhie
Eti	Ugben-eti	Eti	Ikpete
Evwe	Evwro	Evwe	Orji
Ikpamaku	Ikpamaku	Ikpamaku,	Ikpamaku Akanta
Imirhe akpata	Imirhe akpata	imirhe akpata	Irhibo
Irhibo	Irhibo	Irhibo	Irioha
Irieroho	Irioho	Irieroho	Egboronakuwhu
Irrierevwe	Irierevwe	Irrierevwe	Ishakpa,
Ishakpa	Ichakpa	Ishasha, Opuopu	Itetebe
Itetebe	Itetebe	Itetebe	Ekoro
Ivwrevwre	Ivwrevwre	Ivwrevwre	Obukoiyeke
Obukoiyeke	Obukoiyeke	Obukoiyeke	Obherokoko
Obe-okpokpa	Oba-okpokpan	Obe-okpokpa	Obiakpe
Obe-akpe	Obeakpe	Obe-akpe	Ule
Ode	Oluko	Ode	Egiri
Odjigbe	Odjigben	Odjigbe	Ogrishi
Oghriki	Uhimi	Oghriki	Anagbe
Ohahen	Ohahen	Ohehe	Oghighe
Oghighe	Oghighen	Oghigho	Ogba
Okpagha	Okpagha	Okpagha	Onughu
Origbo	Origbon	Origbo	
Owhidide	Kpididen	Owhidide	Owhidide
Owhorome	Owhoroma	Owhoroma	Emiwhororo
Ufierhivwi	Ufierhimi	Ufierhivwi	Ubrubrehivwi
Ugege	Ugege	Ugege	Ugege
Ugboduma	Ugboduma	Ugboduma	Ugboduma
Uho, ufugbu	Who	Uho	Ubo
Utezi	Utezi	Utezi	Ikprogbe
Urierie	Urierie	Urierie	Oda
Urieriewhu	Urieriewhu	Urieriewhu	Ukpereziza
Uware	Uwara	Uwara	Otoro
Umebe	Umeben	Umebe	Ekukuo ofi
Uwara			
Imeben			

CHAPTER FOUR

Evaluation

INTRODUCTION

Urhoboland fundamentally comprises rural communities with few concentrations in Ughelli, Warri, Sapele and Agbarho which can be designated as urban centres. Modern health services are concentrated in these urban areas. In fact, modern hospitals and health centres are only found in Ughelli, Agbarho, Warri, Sapele, Orerokpe, and Eku-a Baptist Hospital which is the most efficient and popular. Thus, the services of doctors, nurses and other health personnel are limited to the urban and semi-urban areas, even though about 90% of the Urhobo population live in the rural areas.

A survey of available Government and Mission Hospitals and Health Centres and their health personnel in Urhoboland indicated that there is significant shortage of manpower, drugs and equipment; thus the provision of health services is grossly inadequate.[1] The realization of these inadequacies has demonstrated the signal role of the involvement of the traditional medicine men and women, midwives and birth attendants, who were hitherto assaulted and were targets of missionary campaigns of vilification, as front line health care personnel . If the health services as indicated by the 1992 research survey are grossly inadequate, a period which was less than nine years to the target year A.D. 2000 when health services were said to be available to all, one can, therefore, surmise the type of health services hitherto provided for the Urhobo by the colonial government and the missions. Against this background, one can understand and assess accurately the contribution of Urhobo traditional medical services to the total well-being of the people.

CONTRIBUTIONS OF URHOBO MEDICINE

Barrenness in Women

One of the areas of human affliction and disease where Urhobo medicine has achieved immense success is barrenness or gynaecological problems. Among the Urhobo, much premium is placed on fecundity. A marriage is considered successful to the extent that the woman gives birth not only to a girl but also a son who will survive and sustain the process of continuity. Thus the signal role of marriage is to satisfy the ambition of the Urhobo man to maintain this continuity of life; for according to Metuh:

> A son's life is the prolongation of the life of his father, his grandfather, his ancestors and the life of the whole lineage. As its numerical strength increases, so does its life force become stronger. Hence, the greatest tragedy that can befall a man and his lineage is for him to die childless.[2]

Cardinal Malula views marriage as a means of assuring the survival of the extended family especially a fruitful marriage. A man or woman who does not procreate is to the African mind, a dead wood which is good for nothing.[3] A married woman can only claim to be a full member of her husband's family only after the birth of a child because it is then that the man is assured of immortality. Hence, Bohannan and Curtin observe:

> Only on the birth of a child does a woman become truly a kinsman in her husband's group. Only on the birth of a child is a man assured of "immortality" of his position in the genealogy of his lineage, or even of security of esteem among the important people of his community. Only on the birth of a grandchild is a man in a position to be truly sure that his name and spirit will live in the history and genealogy of his people.[4]

Such names as *Omonigho* (a child is more important than money), *Omoefe* (a child is wealth), *Aruwevwire* (I have entered the house) and *Etuwevwire* (I have reached home) underscore the vital position a child occupies in Urhobo concept of life.

The practice of polygamy, which Euro-American scholars used to contend that the Africans had no concept of love and that it was a means to subjugate the wives to second-hand position, has its genesis in the African fear of childlessness. The truth, among other reasons, is that Africans, were so preoccupied with the idea of having a child that they adopted the polygamous system of marriage to insure against childlessness, the concept of which is frightening to the Africans. Among the Urhobo, a barren woman is treated with disdain and has no respect among her womenfolk. Ward, commenting on the state of barrenness among the Yoruba women, states:

> Barrenness carries with it a cultural stigma. The barren woman is the most despised creature in the land. There is something deeper in this stigma than the fact that she has not fulfilled her primary function in life. In death, as a rule, her body is thrown into the bush, as it is done with suicides, demented persons and murderers, to be the food of wild animals.[5]

The Urhobo cosmology regarding the causative theory of sickness is personalistic, as Forster has described it. [6] Therefore, the first place of call for women with reproductive problems is the *orhere* (traditional midwives) and *obo* (medicine man/woman). The Urhobo pharmacopoeia is replete with medicine for treating reproductive, obstetric and paediatric diseases. An Urhobo trained in the modern medicine, F. O. Esiri, remarked that Urhobo traditional medical specialists have efficacious gynaecological medicines but that these medicines are wrongly applied, especially as regards the timing. [7] He went on to give an example of how an Urhobo traditional midwife gave a medicine which was meant to ease labour and delivery to a pregnant woman who had the normal pains during pregnancy and not the real labour pain.

It was in recognition of the contributions of the Urhobo traditional midwives and birth attendants that seminars and workshops were being organized for them in Okpe Local Government Council to acquaint them with modern techniques, to encourage them to refer difficult problems to maternity homes and hospitals for proper and quick attention. According to Mrs. Ademenaha, a Senior Nursing Sister in charge of the training programme, the seminars covered such areas as: ante-natal care, environmental sanitation, first stages of labour, nutrition, balanced diet, EPI/ORT, immunization, visit to the hospitals for the study of the sanitary conditions and certain serious cases, women at risk during pregnancy, labour, abortion, anaemia, swollen feet, delayed pregnancy and its associated problems, and prolonged labour. Mr. Mafuru, Principal Health Officer and the Coordinator, Primary Health Care for Okpe Local Government Council emphasized that during the seminars and workshops, the need for both traditional and modern midwives to refer cases was encouraged and that so far, the council had achieved tremendous success in that regard.

Ebo and *irhere* (Medicine men/women and midwives) with their wealth of knowledge in gynaecological, obstetric and paediatric problems and pharmacopoeia have contributed immensely to solving the problem of barrenness among Urhobo women. My research indicated that the bulk of the clientele of medicine men/women who are traditional specialists in gynaecological treatments are more in number among the traditional medical practitioners found in the Urhobo urban centres.

In the treatment of gynaecological problems, the traditional medical practitioner employs both herbal preparations and massaging. If it is discovered that some preternatural forces are responsible for such problems, protective medicine will be prepared. In the latter case, sacrifices may be offered to the ancestors or to the witches to neutralize and render ineffective whatever means they might employ. Protective medicines worn by such women are called *Edaji* and *Amrevwadje*. In addition to the treatment of cases of barrenness, the Urhobo traditional healers also have effective medicines for paediatric cases.

Impotency in Men

Impotency in men may be due to natural or preternatural causations. In the treatment of natural impotency, the *obo* administers herbal preparation with high potency and the condition is reversed. But there are some cases which are due to malformation or development of the male's reproductive organs. In such cases, the *ebo 's* (medicine men/women) medical therapy has its limitation. Wolf has remarked that where sterility has been caused by *Olodumare*, no person on earth, not even the forces of *oogun*, could change his/her fate. [8]

In social/preternatural causation, a witch could seize the potency of the man right from youth or when he has had a wife and children. For instance, a fellow lecturer told me of how his father seized his potency for thirteen years before he could regain it.[9] In a polygamous family, the jealous wife who is a witch could render the husband impotent for her mate. In such a case, the husband can have intercourse with the witch wife but incapable of mating with the second wife. This belief among the Yoruba about the power of witches in rendering a man impotent, is well-articulated by R. Prince:

> It is widely believed that a witch is capable of supernaturally removing a man's penis while he is sleeping and using it to have intercourse with a woman, thereby rendering the man impotent and the woman sterile.[10]

On the other hand, a man may have illicit intercourse with a man's wife. The husband, feeling so aggrieved and contemptuously treated, may prepare *olephe-orha* (retaliatory medicine) to render the adulterer impotent. The preparation of *Olephe* involves the use of some herbs which are very soft and weak *Oghworoma* (a climbing stem) and combining it with the power of the spoken word - *egophiyo*. This category of impotency cannot be cured by western therapy except the *ebo* (medicine men/women) after he/she has duly consulted the *oboepha* (diviner). The prescription, for most part, includes the preparation of *arhare* (potency medicine). In the preparation and administration of *arhare* there is the combination of the power of the herb and the power of the spoken word -*egophiyo*. The herbs used in its preparation are characteristically very tough and hard to break. In all preparation of *arhare*, *egberebo* herb is always used.[11] Bascom also alludes to similar prescription amongst the Yoruba. [12]

Life would have become unbearable for impotent men; but the traditional therapy, which caters for the wholeness of man has helped to make life enjoyable to those so afflicted.

Fractures

The Urhobo believe that cases of fractures are better handled by traditional orthopaedic healers. Fractures which are not complicated are treated, easily without recourse to modern hospitals. Urhobo medicine include antiseptics, *umu ora* and *umu ro sie ihori ne ora*, used to prevent suppuration. The efficiency of the healer in treating complicated fracture is attested to by many scholars. Rt. Rev. S. N. Ezeanya, doubtful though he is about the efficacy of traditional medicine, gives an example of a fractured ankle which the hospital could not handle but was effectively taken care of by a bone-setter. As he argues the case:

> They took the student home to a bone-setter who broke the bone again and reset it. After a few weeks, the young man returned to school with a normal leg so well treated that it was not possible to know which of his legs was the fractured one.[13]

He only attributes the success of fractured bones which do not pierce the body to bone-setters but doubts their ability to treat complicated fractures. He believes that bone-setters have no antiseptic. Hence he contends that such sores go septic.

Nobody doubts Ezeanya's assertion because in both orthodox and traditional medicine, any mismanaged sores usually go septic. The fact is that there are effective natural antiseptics in traditional medicine. Dopamu attests to the efficacy of osteopathic medicine and the efficiency displayed by the bone–setters. He opines that:

> Some people in my village had a ghastly motor accident on their way to the village. Many of them had complex fractures such as should have resulted in amputation in the hospital, but they were taken to *Egun*, bone-setter at Abeokuta. They were successfully treated and discharged within five months.[14]

My research revealed that this is an area where there is referral between the traditional bone-setters and the modern hospitals. According to Oghenesivwohwo of Ekrokpe, the first reaction of relatives of patients with complex fractures among the Urhobo is to take the patient to modern hospital to treat the wounds after which the aspect of bone-setting is brought to them. In most cases, the orthodox doctors are unaware of the procedure.

Bone-setting is, in most cases, regarded as heirloom whose knowledge is never transmitted to anybody outside the family. Attempts usually made to procure such medicines have met with serious disappointment.[15] Mr. Akpovwovwo, a bone-setter at Agbarho and Mr. Onorehwovo of Eboh-Orogun also narrated the different efforts made by orthodox doctors and researchers including myself to purchase the medicine. Mr. Onorohwovo specifically mentioned several visitations he had got from medical doctors at Eku and Igbobi Hospitals after he had successfully treated a patient who could not be treated in these modern hospitals. In spite of all persuasions and offering of substantial sum of money by the medical doctors, Mr. Onorohwovo blatantly refused.[16] The rareness of amputants in the Urhobo societies is attributed to the existence of osteopathic medicines and the efficiency of the Urhobo bone-setters.

My interview with Mr. Oko, an Abraka man with amputated leg revealed that the leg was amputated when he was in the army. He lamented the amputation and remarked that if he were at home, (Abraka) the leg would not have been amputated.[17] One is often tempted to indict the governments especially the states for not showing sufficient encouragement in the development of traditional medicine. Such efficient bone-setters should be encouraged to practise in government hospitals as specialists in their own field. Through this means, the knowledge of such medicine will be gradually revealed. Secondly, the government should encourage traditional healers with such efficacious medicine to register them with her and their patents duly accorded them and should be paid royalty on subsequent productions.

Treatment of Psychosocial and Supernatural Diseases

It has been discovered that there is an intimate relationship between the practice of medicine and culture. I have discussed Payer's investigation on the correlation between culture and the practice of western medicine among the German, French, English and American, peoples with almost the same life expectancy. From his research, he concluded that there is much correlation between culture and practice of western medicine. In the same vein among the Urhobo, there is inherent relationship between the practice of medicine and culture. As I have mentioned in chapter four, there are diseases within the psychosocial and supernatural levels that cannot be cured by orthodox medicine.

Africans trained in western medicine often advise patients whose diseases appear to have social/preternatural or supernatural causative background, to seek traditional treatment. It is explicit that in Urhobo there are diseases which can only be cured through traditional medication. Thus there are instances according to Idowu when relatives of patients admitted to hospital smuggled in for them medicine obtained from traditional doctor"[18] Ejizu clearly illustrates with two cases of forceful removal of patients from hospitals, after abortive attempts to secure cure, to traditional healers where cure was effected within appreciable periods. [19]

The perennial shortage of medical personnel, drugs and equipment, the distance of many of the Urhobo health care consumers from hospitals, dispensaries, health centres, maternity homes and other government and mission health institutions coupled with the proved efficacy of traditional medicine has given traditional medicine a pride of place in the Urhobo health care delivery system. It has thus contributed immensely to the restoration, preservation and enhancement of life among the Urhobo. Apart from these diseases, the Urhobo also believe that diseases like asthma, epilepsy, paralysis, stroke, diabetes, and fracture are better handled and treated by traditional medicine. The existence and continuity of traditional medicine amid the tremendous medical technology and the continued patronage of the system by both literate and illiterate, Christians, Moslems, the rich and the poor is an affirmation of the efficacy of traditional medicine and its contribution to the Urhobo health care system.

DEFECTS OF URHOBO MEDICINE

Every medical system has its strong and weak points. It is therefore, not surprising that Urhobo medical practice has its strong and weak points. I have discussed the strong points of Urhobo medicine above. It is worthy of note that orthodox medicine with its high technological advancement has its merits and demerits. In this section, the allegations levied against Urhobo traditional medicine will be examined.

Claims to Ability to Cure All Types of Ailments

Urhobo medical practitioners are accused of claiming to be adepts in the treatment of all kinds of ailments whether naturally or supernaturally caused. Among the Urhobo healers, some lay claim to be generalists in an attempt to make quick money from patients. Mr. Okohwake of Arhavwarien did not doubt the allegation but claimed that there were specialists in bone-setting, paralysis, mental troubles, and epilepsy; that these diseases were usually referred to them by both medicine men/women and ordinary people who knew them.[20] These specialists view their medicament as a heirloom whose knowledge they feel is recondite and mysterious to others outside the family. These specialists have, in most cases, proved the efficacy of their medicine. There is an element of truth in the allegation because nobody doubts the presence of charlatans in the system.

This claim may be due to the healer's inability to diagnose properly the diseases, as happens at times in orthodox diagnostic procedure. But after some ineffective treatment, such patients are usually referred to the specialist or their relatives forcefully withdraw them from the hands of the healers, as sometimes occurs in modern hospitals. Other allegations levelled against Urhobo traditional medicine practitioners include, secrecy, problem of over-dosage and operating in insanitary conditions.

Secrecy

Every profession has its rules and regulations which guide its members. These rules and regulations may be referred to as the ethics of such profession. The orthodox medical profession is no exemption. For instance, the Hippocratic oath forbids members of the profession from divulging their patients' secrets to non-members. But such secrets or problems might be discussed among members in an attempt to find solutions to them.

Urhobo medicine as a profession is distinct. Among its members, secrecy is eschewed. There is constant exchange of ideas relating to the knowledge, preparation and application of drugs. This exchange of ideas is possible because of the establishment of traditional healers' associations at the local level. All these local bodies are affiliated to Urhobo Association of Traditional Healers.[21] Referral is, therefore, a commonplace experience among them because they are aware of who possesses what medicine. In their meetings, there is always some exchange of ideas and discussion of problems facing them. The coming together of the local associations and their demand for recognition by state and federal governments culminated in the formation of the Nigerian Council of Traditional Medical Practitioners whose first chairman was Chief Abimbola Sodipe.[22]

However, like every other profession, secrecy is an aspect of their ethics. The medicine men view their profession as sacred. They believe that sacred things should only be divulged to the sacred and initiated members, but not to the uninitiated. It is after the initiation ritual that the new entrant is, as of right, qualified to receive such revelation. The maintenance of secrecy assists in the regulation of the number of entrants into the profession; consequently the number of the group is restricted through the introduction of fees to be paid before learning the secrets.

The Urhobo medicine men differ from the Yoruba healers whom Maclean describes as always ready to discuss their medicine with a researcher who displays sympathetic understanding.[23] But they are similar to Dopamu's interviewees, who viewed divulging the secret of their medicine as losing their main source of livelihood.[24] The level of awareness of the Urhobo healers is so low that none of them, I interviewed, ever discussed a single medicine and the disease it cures. They viewed the researcher as a potential medicine man who was collecting their medicine under the guise of carrying out research.

Receipt of Money before the Revelation of Medicine

African medicine men are also accused of receiving money before the revelation of their medicine. In Urhobo, the payment of money is considered as one factor which they believe ensures the efficacy and value of the medicine. Some fathers even before they reveal medicine to their children demand the payment of some money. In cases where the son cannot provide the money, the father himself gives the required amount to him who will in turn give it back to him as a token fee. Among the Yoruba, it is a common practice and belief that medicine in which payment is not made is always carelessly placed and not valued. This philosophy is true with the Urhobo who believe that *Obo-wo vwori ro da we ero oye we vwa erote* (it is what you treasure that you jealously guard.) However, there are also fathers who bequeath their medicine to their children as a means of providing means of livelihood for them; just as a father consciously trains his children to any level of education.

Overdosage

The problem of overdosage is another accusation levelled against traditional medicine. The proponents of this view argue that the problem of overdosage is consequent upon the African lack of anatomic and physiological knowledge. Ezeanya's viewpoint is again a representative example of this group. He contends that:

> The medicine man does not have instruments with which to measure the temperature and the heartbeats. Nor has he the instruments with which to examine delicate organs like the eyes and ear. The result is that in many cases, treatment which is given is altogether out of proportion to the need and capacity of patient's body. The consequence often is that complications set in as a result of overdosage or the administration of wrong drug for a particular sickness.[25]

Urhobo medical knowledge is experiential and not experimental but the Urhobo healer is not as naive as Ezeanya has presented him. Ezeanya fails to realize that African healers undergo a long period of tutelage under experienced and elderly healers. The period of apprenticeship varies from three to seven years. During the period, the neophyte acquires what is necessary in the medical science.

Furthermore, the problem of overdosage, if it is there at all, is not peculiar to Urhobo healers. Some patients out of the urge to get cured of their ailments take overdose. This occurs both in orthodox and traditional medicines. However, Ezeanya's view is countered by Gilles Bibeau et. al. who accused those who deny traditional healers the possession of an organized body of anatomic and physiological knowledge. Gilles Bibeau and others concede this knowledge to the healers. They believe that the way the traditional healers administer remedies and especially the location of incision indicates their knowledge of the relationship between the head, the heart and their view about blood circulation. That the specialized and large pharmacopeia which they use for the control of the body's function even attests to it.[26] As regards overdosage, Gilles Bibeau et.al. contend:

> Some healers measure out dosage in cups rather than in teaspoon; they know that an overdosage leads to poisoning and that an insufficient dose is tantamount to lack of therapy; they take into account the characteristics of the patients—age and height, of the illness itself either mild (incipient), chronic, or serious and of the contents both of the treatment and of the remedy (rapid, slow, violent).[27]

In the same vein, Abayomi Sofowora's remarks that many traditional healers specify dosage, even using terms like teaspoonful and so on and varying the dose according to the age of the patients,[28] corroborates the viewpoint of Gilles Bibeau et.al.

Traditional healers, Okpako [29] and Umukoro,[30] Madam Oti, opined that the accusation of overdosage against traditional medicine is due to the campaign of vilification mounted by the western trained doctors. They contended that most traditional medicine are concocted from herbs which are, in most part, used as vegetable and hardly could one take an overdose of these vegetables. Oguakwa specifically argues that the toxicity of herbal medicine is greatly mitigated through boiling and the addition of extracts of other roots and oil. Thus Oguakwa asserts:

> When he prepares a new medicine with a new herb, he dilutes it with palm oil and gives a portion of it to a dog for testing purposes because it is believed that what kills a dog can also kill a human being. Furthermore, the issue of overdose is well-known to an Africanist who purposely adds the extracts of certain other roots into some prepared medicines so that if a patient takes an overdose of it either deliberately or mistakingly, he vomits automatically.[31]

The problem of overdosage, the Urhobo healers argued, was an attempt to call a dog a bad name so that it could be hanged.

Insanitary Condition

The problem of insanitary condition in which healers operate is a serious problem which Urhobo healers are still grappling with. Many of the healers' houses, except Mume who has a modern tradomedical hospital, often have offensive odours oozing from rotten *materia medica* safely stored in some parts of the room. At times, it could be oozing from gin and blood of victims offered to his medical paraphernalia or used for the preparation of remedies. The healers have no effective preservative methods. Many of the leaves, roots and other materials for medical preparations are stored in the house to provide ready materials. So long as the healers lack effective preservative methods of their *materia medica*, this problem will continue to linger on.

Furthermore, most healers prepare some medicine without due regard to rules of hygiene. In some cases, the mortar used for pounding medicine is not properly washed before and after use. In serving the drinks presented by the hospitable healer/patient, the same cup/glass is used for everybody; the nature of the diseases of the different patients notwithstanding. Arubalueze's research among the lgbo healers also confirms this argument. He remarks that:

> Where we were served palm wine and dry gin, popularly called "hot drink" we were in most cases provided with common cups to drink in turn. In fact, we had enough evidence to confirm the impression that most of our traditionalists perform under very poor hygienic conditions.[32]

Western orthodox medicine, which is the summation of human medical heritage from diverse cultures, nationalities, and races,[33] was also bedevilled with the problem of insanitary conditions. The history of medicine in Victorian England has revealed that progress in medicine was slow and gradual. Before Lister, what was common practice in English hospitals was unhygienic and deplorable. For instance, in 1862 it was being argued that bandages and instruments used for the treatment of gangrenous wounds ought not, if possible, be used a second time. It was being considered whether bandages, linen or clothing should be kept in rooms where infected patients were lying.[34] It was later that Lister discovered that germs were the main cause of the suppuration of sores or fractures. In his paper on *The Antiseptic Principle in the Practice of Surgery*, he advocated cleanliness and the maintenance of rules of hygiene in hospitals.[35] Thus the sanitary condition of modern hospitals has its provenance in Lister's learned advocacy.

To overcome the problem of insanitary conditions of Urhobo healers, the federal, state and local governments should have arms of traditional medicine. Here, the activities of the healers will be coordinated by medical officers and other health personnel. These health personnel should faithfully report the achievement and failures of traditional healers. Secondly, the health personnel should inculcate simple rules and regulations of hygiene on the healers. Seminars and workshops should be organized for them during which period they should be given opportunity to visit hospital to see for themselves the sanitary nature of the hospitals and other health service centres. Thirdly, a more comprehensive means of preserving the various herbs should be worked out by the government. Preferably, botanical gardens should be developed where some of the medicinal plants should be planted and made readily available for the healers. The various governments should come up with positive measures aimed at improving traditional medicine. By incorporating the traditional healers into the orthodox medical system, they will of necessity abandon their insanitary nature and appreciate the need for the maintenance of rules of hygiene. It is through this means that in no distant future, there will be Urhobo (African) Medical Renaissance. Africa, like China, would then emerge with a medical system adoptable all over the world.

CHAPTER FIVE

Summary and Conclusion

SUMMARY

Urhobo medicine is a distinct medical system which is at variance, in some aspects, with modern orthodox medical system. The difference emanates from the difference in the cosmologies in which they are practised. These worldviews underline the people's perception of disease and their treatment modalities. Hence it has been argued that the understanding of the Urhobo medicine warrants a thorough understanding of the Urhobo cosmology. The inability of the early anthropologists, ethnologists and missionaries to understand Urhobo medicine and the subsequent utilization of derogatory terms to describe the medical system and its practitioner emerged from errors of judgement and interpretation. Thus, they erroneously used their culture lens, based on the scientific model, to judge the Urhobo worldview which is essentially religious.

Egophiyo (incantations or words of intention) and rituals are characteristic features of Urhobo medicine. This is based on the people's belief that man as a finite being, cannot on his own achieve success without the intervention of the supernatural powers, especially *Oghene, esemo* and *iniemo.* Consequently, among the Urhobo, an unconsecrated medicine is thought inefficacious. Moreover, the Urhobo believe that all objects are imbued with life force which is the quintessence of the thing itself. These natural powers/forces as such could only be activated and set in motion through the use of *egophiyo* by the *obo.* This esoteric knowledge possessed by the *obo* is acquired during training. *Egophiyo,* therefore, potentates and finally effectuates the needed cure. This is why we assert that the *obo's* approach to disease among the Urhobo is essentially holistic. The *obo* reaches the different levels of the Urhobo perception of the aetiology of diseases in all his treatment. This is the benefit of Urhobo medicine over modern medicine. Although *egophiyo* (incantations) and rituals in Urhobo medicine may be meaningless to the westerner but they are integral part and even therapeutic in Urhobo medical system especially in diseases caused preternaturally and supernaturally. Thus among the Urhobo, emphasis is placed on the maintenance of wholesome personal relations with the family, community and the supersensible realities.

We have discovered that the Urhobo medical practitioners were the target of the missionary campaigns of vilification. They were thus dubbed witch-doctor, hunter and were viewed as embodiment and propagators of the vilest values. But from the foregoing, it has been shown that these accusations were baseless and false. The proponents of the view that traditional medicine and its practitioners would gradually disappear as modern medicine develops and advances technologically, have also been proved wrong.

Schwartz[1], Maclean[2], Janzen[3], Press[4] and Twumasi[5] have asserted that the appearance of modern medicine and its interaction with the traditional medical system does not portend the disappearance of the latter. Harrison, on the other hand, has rightly observed that:

> Much to the chagrin of some and to the amazement of others, native doctors in Nigeria will not go away, fade away or cease to practise. Healers, worldwide, are rather conservative. They are a privileged class, have status and wield power, both secular and profane.[6]

The Urhobo medicine is practised in a culture that is dynamic and growing more complex daily. The Christians, elites and agnostics have been so brainwashed that they decry any modicum of goodness in traditional medicine. Their attitudes become more vicious because of the various rituals involved in the system. From the analysis, it is evident that some of these rituals are inherent in the system; others may have been introduced into it by the Urhobo professionals to conceal their efficacious therapeutic remedies from the curious eyes of their patients and relatives. It has been opined that the extrinsic rituals could be mitigated while those intrinsic to the Urhobo medical system, whose performance renders not only Urhobo therapy effective but also modern medicines, should be encouraged, and that these intrinsic rituals are the distinct characteristics of Urhobo medicine.

Urhobo elites, Christians and agnostics have to re-educate themselves that Urhobo medicine really works, as against the negative, unprogressive and apathetic attitude of the antagonists of Urhobo medicine. Walter Rodney has rightly observed that it is among the educated Africans we find the most alienated.[7] Frantz Fanon has summoned the Africans to divest themselves of colonial trappings and indoctrination which have estranged them from developing and advancing their culture. As Fanon puts it:

> Come, then, comrades; it would be as well to decide at once to change our ways. We must shake off the heavy darkness in which we were plunged, and leave it behind. The new day which is already at hand must find us firm, prudent and resolute.[8]

It is with this resolute determination to reassess and develop our culture that the Urhobo medicine will advance.

CONCLUSION

This work has provided Urhobo pharmacopoeia. From the Urhobo perspective, this work is seminal in the sense that this is the first attempt to pry into Urhobo medicine. With this work, the existing gap between Urhobo and other Nigerian peoples, who have developed their pharmacopoeia, has been bridged. We do not in the least, pretend that this work is exhaustive. We have only ventured to assert that it will, to some extent, serve as a source material for the pharmacological analysis of Urhobo medicine.

The Urhobo medicine and its practitioner need improvement if the Urhobo are to achieve effective health delivery system, which is at present eluding them. The bulk of the Urhobo live in the rural areas where effective modern medical system is lacking. To achieve effective health care system, the *ebo* who are ubiquitous in every Urhobo village must be integrated into the medical system.

Ademuwagun has suggested seven points why the services of the *ebo* are indispensable. He opines that:

(i)   traditional healers could easily fill the vacuum in health care created by the shortage of health personnel and the high cost of training modern health workers;

(ii)   in their treatment techniques, traditional healers demonstrate astute approach to human ecology and health;

(iii)   they are of the same culture with their patients, sharing common beliefs, values and symbols of communication;

(iv)   they have developed traditional skills in dispensing curative, preventive and rehabilitative care;

(v)   they are efficient in some aspects of psychosomatic medicine and in using local herbs, roots and bark for psychosomatic therapy;

(vi)   they are not disturbed by problem of inadequate transportation in rural areas;

(vii)   they are skilful in interpersonal relations, including counselling with sympathy, identification and concern.[9]

Among the Urhobo, attempt is being made to re-educate the *ebo* in some techniques in modern medicine. For instance, in Okpe Local Government Council, the signal role of the traditional medical personnel in the health care system has been realized. Their deficiencies are being catered for by organizing seminars and workshops for them. During the seminars, they are taught referral procedures and its need, improved sanitary conditions and other related issues.[10]

A better utilization of Urhobo traditional medicine requires a good knowledge of the various herbs and the diseases they treat. Unfortunately, the professionals who have the esoteric knowledge of Urhobo medicine are ageing and dying away. If immediate and positive step is not taken, to record the knowledge from them, this aspect of the Urhobo heritage might finally disappear into oblivion. We strongly suggest therefore that:

(i)   a highly potent and efficacious medicine like the arthritis medicine which Mr. Eyimofe refused to divulge, needs a thorough study by the government, and to encourage such people to reveal the knowledge to doctors as additional remedy for the treatment of arthritis;

(ii)   such highly effective medicine could be registered with the government and royalty duly paid to them for any production; and

(iii)   a team of government-sponsored pharmacological students and scholars should visit the *ebo* to acquire such medicine for laboratory analysis.

A new development which is posing a serious threat to the practice of Urhobo medicine is the rate of deforestation and large scale annual bush burning. Deforestation has reduced immensely Urhobo medicinal plants. Consequently, trees whose barks, roots, or leaves are potent for therapeutic purposes are becoming extinct. Such medicines will of necessity become obsolete and gradually fall into a state of desuetude from the Urhobo pharmacopoeia. Added to the deforestation is the annual indiscriminate bush burning. Like deforestation, bush burning has contributed greatly to the disappearance of some herbs which are highly medicinal.

To arrest the situation, federal and state governments as well as local government councils should declare expanses of land as forest reserves. Secondly, they should encourage the establishment of botanical gardens where highly potent medicinal plants should be planted after such medicinal plants have been duly analyzed pharmacologically. Bush burners should be dealt with seriously by instituting stringent penalty against them.

In conclusion, the Urhobo elites, Christians and agnostics are called upon to note what Peter Berger calls "alternation". By alternation, Peter Berger calls on humanity to reassess and attempt a critical evaluation of the various trends in world history. This critical evaluation, he argues, will lead to the realization of something radically different from what had been previously taken for granted.[11] Against the old concepts about Urhobo medicines, the Urhobo people will discover also that there are some diseases which modern medicine cannot cure but are effectively cured by Urhobo medicine, and that diseases are becoming resistant to modern synthetic medicine. There is, therefore, popular advocacy for the use of medicinal plants. This alternation will enable Urhobo medicine to contribute its quota to medicine in general and particularly to the realization of "Health For All" in Urhobo land.

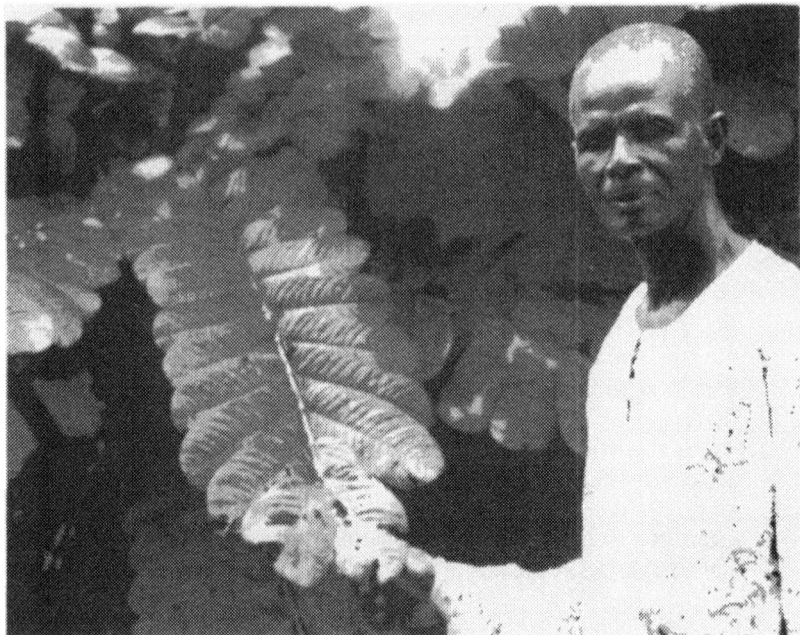

Amoke / Okekpobevwerhe

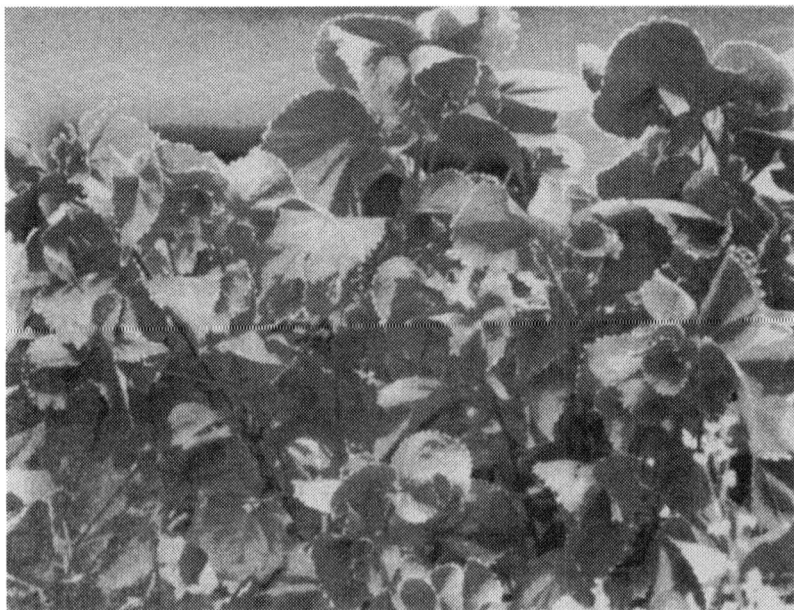

Croton

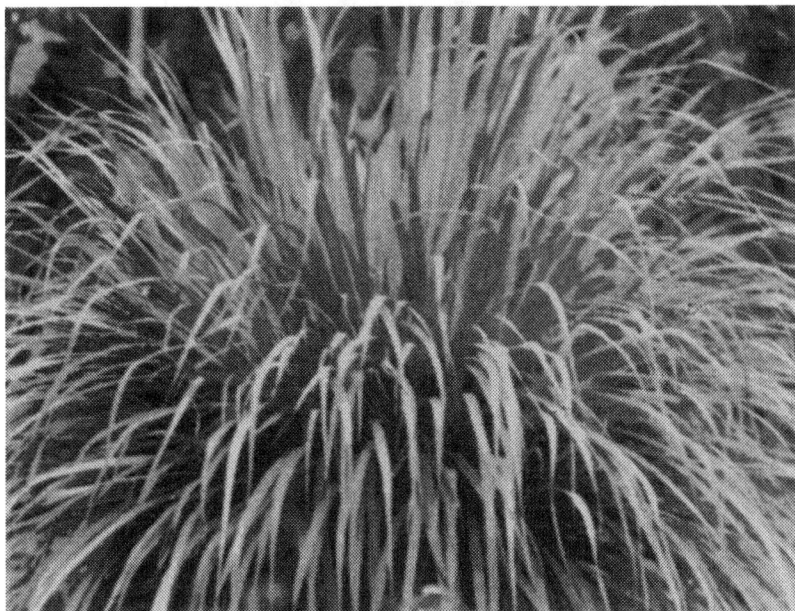

Lemon Grass
Urhobo Name - *Obeitie*
Botanical Name - *Cymbopogon*

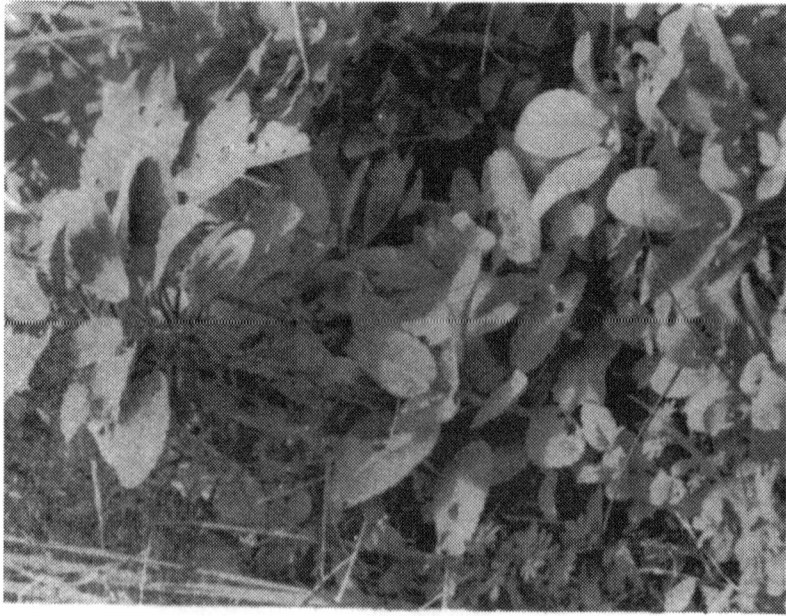

Scent Leaves
Urhobo Name - *Eran*
Botanical Name - *Ocimum basilicum*

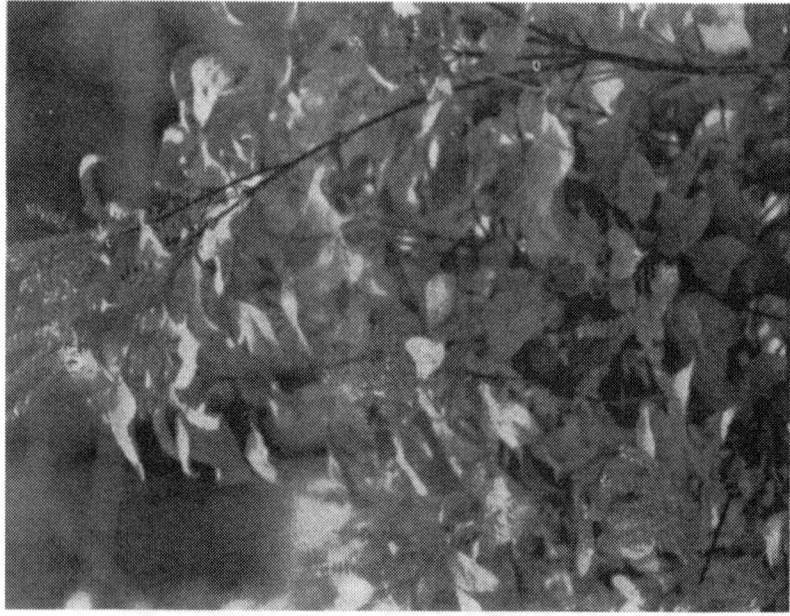

Urhobo Name - *Obekpokpa*
Botanical Name - *Bryophillum*

Appendix 1

1992 research Survey of Government and Mission Health Service Centres in Urhoboland.

No.	Local Government Area	No. of Government Hospitals	No. of Mission Hospitals	No. of Health Centres	No. of Health Personnel
1.	Ethiope East Isiokolo	-	1	-	200
2.	Ethiope West Ogharefe	-	-	4	10
3.	Okpe, Orerokpe	2	-	10	25
4.	Sapele Sapele	1 -	- -	6 -	18 -
5.	Ughelli North, Ughelli	1	-	9	20
6.	Ughelli South, Otu Jeremi	1	-	8	18

Private Health Service Centres in Urhoboland.

Towns	No. of Health Service Centres	No. of Workers
Abraka	2	10
Agbarho	1	5
Sapele	10	50
Oghara	-	-
Idjerhe	-	-
Ughelli	9 including Maternity Homes	20
Warri	20 including Maternity Homes	400

Appendix 11

Federal Republic of Nigeria 1991 Population Census by Rank, Delta State

(Provision Results)

S/N	L.G.A. Name	Males	Females	Males
*1.	Okpe	132,722	128,708	261,430
*2.	Warri South	109,818	103,458	213,276
3.	Ndokwa West	88,466	94,784	183,250
*4.	Ugheli North	77,807	83,350	16,157
5.	Burutu North	85,352	75,093	160,445
6.	Isoko South	69,890	72,773	142,663
*7.	Sapele South	71,198	70,043	141,241
8.	Bomadi South	70,100	70,336	140,436
9.	Isoko North	64,199	69,533	133,732
*10.	Ughelli South	60,243	71,048	131,291
11.	Ika South	63,674	56,261	129,932
12.	Oshimili South	61,582	61,021	122,603
13.	Aniocha South	56,003	56,395	112,603
14.	Ika North East	52,820	57,696	110,516
*15.	Ethiope East	52,173	56,530	108,703
*16.	Ethiope West	50,275	50,210	101,585
17.	Warri North	44,598	42,846	87,444
18.	Ndokwa East	34,908	37,773	72,681
19.	Aniocha North	27,280	28,115	55,395
	Total	1,273,208	1,296,973	2,570,181

*The six Urhobo Local Government Areas. Apart from these, Warri South Local Government Area is made up of the Urhobo, Izon and Itsekiri

Notes and References

Chapter One pp: 1-19

1. J. U. Oguakwa "Authenticity of African Traditional Medicine: Validity and Provocative Consequences: A New Philosophical Dimension in Traditional Medicine" A Paper Presented at the International Workshop on "African Philosophy in a Scientific and Technological Age", Dept. of Philosophy, University of Nigeria, Nsukka, December 13-16, 1990, p. 2.

2. J. O. Kokwora, *Medicinal Plants in East Africa,* (Nairobi: East African Literature Bureau, 1976), p. 2.

3. M. M. Iwu. *Traditional Igbo Medicine.* Report of a Project Sponsored by the Institute of African Studies, University of Nigeria, Nsukka, 1981.

4. I. U. W. Osisiogu. "Some Notes on African's Drug Plant Heritage" in *Ikenga,* Vol. 1, No. 2, July (1972), p. 84.

5. Quoted in M. M. Iwu: *Traditional Igbo Medicine, Op. cit.* p. 33.

6. G. W. Harley. *Native African Medicine with Special Reference to Its Practice in the Mano Tribe of Liberia,* (London: Frank Cass, 1970), p. 137.

7. A. Smith of Cyprus. *A Contribution to South African Materia Medica* (Lovedale: South Africa, 1988), p. 5.

8. J. A. A. Ayoade "Concept of Inner Essence in Yoruba Traditional Medicine" in *African Therapeutic Systems,* (ed. by). Z. A. Ademuwagun *et.al.* by (Massachusetts: Crossroads Press, 1979), p. 53.

9. A. Alland (Jr.). *Adaptation in Cultural Evolution: An approach to medical anthropology* (New York: Columbia University Press, 1970), p. 127.

10. J. O. Mume, (n.d.) *Traditional Medicine in Nigeria.* (Agbarho: Jom Nature Cure Centre), p. 29f.

11. J. U. Oguakwa, "Authenticity of African Traditional Medicine: Validity and Provocative Consequence: A New Philosophical Dimension in Traditional Medicine, *Op. cit,* p. 1.

12. B. Oliver, *Medicinal Plants in Nigeria,* (Ibadan: The Nigeria College of Arts, Science & Technology, 1960), p. 2.

13. A Alland (Jr.). *Adaptation in Cultural Evolution: An approach to medical anthropology, Op. cit.,* p. 127.

14.   P.A. Dopamu, "Health and Healing within the Traditional African Religious Context" in *ORITA*, Vol. 17, No 2, Dec. (1985), p. 67.

15.   C. Nze, "Logic in African Charm Medicine" in *The Nigerian Journal of Social Studies*, Vol. 4, No.1, (1987), p. 21.

16.   T. Winterbottom. *An Account of the Native Africans in the Neighbourhood of Sierra Leone*, Vol. II, (London: Frank Cass, 1969), p. 4.

17.   P.A. Dopamu, "Health and Healing within the Traditional African Religious Context" in *ORITA*, (1985), *Op. cit.*, p. 68.

18.   T. Winterbottom. *An Account of the Native Africans in the Neighbourhood of Sierra Leone; Op. cit.*, p. 8. Laciany Keita has argued that systematic analysis of historical research of African Cultural History, indicates that the Ancient Egyptian Civilization is fundamentally African and that the first world culture to be involved in systematic appraisal of the world was African — the Africans of Ancient Egypt, that the philosophers and scientists of yesteryears and today are essentially borrowers (See L. Keita , "The African Philosophical Tradition" in *African Philosophy*, (ed.) Richard Wright, (Lanham MD: University Press of America, 1984), p. 8.

19.   M. M. Iwu, "Symbolism and Selectivity in *Traditional African Medicine*" A lecture delivered by the Winner of Vice-Chancellor's Research Leadership Prize for 1987, University of Nigeria, Nsukka, Jan. 12, 1989, p. 8.

20.   T. Winterbottom, *An Account of the Native Africans in the Neighbourhood of Sierra Leone, Op. cit.*, p 9.

21.   O. Nduka, "Rationality and Technological Development": A Paper Presented at the 1964 Silver Jubilee of the Dept. of Philosophy, U. N. N., pp. 3 & 4.

22.   A. J. Youngson, *The Scientific Revolution in Victorian Medicine*, (New York: Homes and Mever Publishers, 1971), p. 212.

23.   D. Lamb, *The Africans: Encounter from Sudan to the Cape*, (London: 1986), p. 140. Also see I. Mbafo, *Towards a Mature African Christianity*, (Enugu: Fourth Dimension, 1989), p. 101. J. Nkpong, "Contextualizing Theological Education in West African" in *African Christian Studies*, (Nairobi, September, 1989), p. 69.

24.   Ngugi Wa Thiong'O, *Decolonizing the Mind*, (London: Currey Press, 1986), p.4.

25.   W. Rodney, *How Europe Underdeveloped Africa*, (Da Es Salaam: Tanzania, 1972), pp. 99-197.

26.   I. V. Sertima. Cited by Ngugi Wa Thiong' O. *Decolonizing the Mind*, Also see G. O. Ehusani, *An Afro-Christian Vision*: "Ozovehe" (Ibadan: Ambassador Publications, 1992), pp. 19 & 35.

27.   Walter L. Williams, *Black Americans and the Evangelization of Africa*: 1877-1900, (Wisconsin: University of Wisconsin Press, 1982), pp. 6 & 7.

28.   Hegel, *The Philosophy of History*, (New York: Dover, 1956), pp. 91-99.

29.   Walter Rodney, *How Europe Underdeveloped Africa* (Dar-es-Salaam; Tanzania Publishing House, 1972), Op. cit, p. 157; G. O. Ehusani, *An Afro-Christian Vision*, p. 82.

30.   G. Guest, *The March of Civilization*, (London: G. Bell and Sons, 1961), p. 105f.

31.   A. Fajana and B. J. Biggs, *Nigeria in History*, (Ibadan: Longman, 1964), p. 156.

32.   E. G. Parrinder, *African Traditional Religion*, (London: S.C.M. 1969), p.156.

33.   E. I. Metuh, "African Traditional Medicine and Healing: A Theological and Pastoral Reappraisal" in *LUCERNA*, Jan.- June (1985) Vol. 6, No. 1, p. 5.

34.   E. I. Metuh, *African Religions in Western Conceptual Schemes*, (Ibadan: Pastoral Institute, Bodija, 1985), p. 162.

35.   P. A. Dopamu, *"Health and Healing within the Traditional African Religious Context"*, p. 67.

36.   E. B. Idowu, *African Traditional Religion: A Definition*, (London: S. C. M. 1973), p. 197.

37.   J. O. Mume, *Traditional Medicine in Nigeria*, (Agbarho: Jom Curative Centre (n.d.), p. 27.

38.   A. Sofowora, *Medicinal Plants and Traditional Medicine in Africa*. (Ibadan: Spectrum Books, 1984), p. 21.

39.   J. O. Awolalu and P. A. Dopamu, *West African Traditional Religion*: (Ibadan: Onibonoje Press, 1979), p. 240.

40.   P. A Dopamu, *"Yoruba Magic and Medicine and Their Relevance for Today"* in *Religions* (NASR), p.3.

41.   *Ibid*. p. 3.

42.   Interview with Edafiadjeka Mark on June 21, 1990, Agwe 67.

43.   Una Maclean, *Magical Medicine: A Nigerian case study*, p. 13.

44.   R. R. Marret, "Magic" in Encyclopaedia of Religion and Ethics (ed. by James Hastings), (Edinburgh: T & T Clark, 1971), Vol. 8, p. 235.

45.   A Shorter, *African Culture and the Christian Church,* (London: Geoffrey Chapman, 1973), p. 131.

46.   J.A.A. Ayoade, "The Concept of Inner Essence in Yoruba Traditional Medicine" in *African Therapeutic Systems,* (ed. by Z. A. Ademuwagun, J.A.A. Ayoade *et.al.*) (Massachusetts: Crossroad Press, 1979), Op. cit., pp. 51 & 52.

47.   M. Oduyoye, "The Medicine man, The Magician and The Wise Man" in *Traditional Religion in West Africa,* (ed. by), A. A. Adegbola, (Ibadan: Daystar, 1983), p. 65.

48.   *Ibid.* p. 67.

49.   J. U. Oguakwa, "Authenticity of African Traditional Medicine: Validity and Provocative Consequences: A New Philosophical Dimension in Traditional Medicine", Op. cit. p. 5f.

50.   V. Omuabor, "Face to Face with Juju Man" in *African Concord,* Vol. 38, April (1987), p.14.

51.   J. U. Oguakwa, "Authenticity of African Traditional Medicine" *Op. cit.* p.6.

52.   N. Azikiwe, *Renanscent Africa,* (London: Frank Case, 1968), p. 142.

53.   *Ibid.* p.6.

54.   A. Shorter. *African Culture and the Christian Church,* (London: Geoffrey Chapman, 1973, p. 129.

55.   E.G. Parrinder, *African Traditional Religion,* (London: Shaldon Press, 1975, 3rd ed.) p. 133.

56.   J.O. Awolalu and P.A. Dopamu, *West African Traditional Religion.* (Ibadan: Onibonoje Press, 1979), p. 246.

57.   P.A. Dopamu, "The Reality of Isasi, Apata, Ironsi and Efun as Forces of Evil" *Unpublished Article,* 1987, p. 246,61.

58.   C.C. Achebe, *The World of the Ogbanje,* (Enugu: Fourth Dimension, 1986), p. 10.

59.   O.U. Kalu, Religion, Medicine and Healing in Nigeria. A keynote Review at the Third Annual Workshop organized by the Department of Religion, University of Ife, Ile-Ife, (n.d.), p. 4.

60. M. M. Iwu, "Symbolism and Selectivity in Traditional African Medicine". A Lecture Delivered by the Winner of Vice-Chancellor's Research Leadership Prize for 1987, University of Nigeria, Nsukka, January 12, 1989, *Op. cit.* p. 3.

61. M. Gelfand, *Medicine and Custom in Africa.* (Edinburgh & London: E.S Livingstone, 1964), p. 137.

62. M. Gelfand, *The African Witch,* (Edinburgh & London: E.S Livingstone, 1967).

63. J. S. Mbiti, *African Religions and Philosophy,* (London: Heinemann, 1969), p. 170.

64. J. U. Oguakwa, "Authenticity of African Traditional Medicine: Validity and Perspective, Consequences; A New Philosophical Dimension in Traditional Medicine". *Op. cit.* p. 4.

65. G. Bibeau *et. al. Traditional Medicine in Zaire: Present and Potential Contribution to the Health Service.* (Ottawa: International Development Centre, 1980), p. 14.

66. Z.A. Ademuwagun, "Problem and Prospect of Legitimatizing Aspects of Traditional Health Care Systems and Methods with Modern Medical Therapy" in *African Therapeutic Systems,* p. 161.

67. C.I. Ejizu, "Healing as Wholeness: The Igbo Experience" in *Africana Marburgeogia.* (ed. by I.T. Hackett), Vol. 129, (1988), p.12.

68. E.E. Evans-Pritchard, *The Theories of Primitive Religion,* (Oxford: Clarendon Press, 1965), p.7.

69. N. Ezeabasili, *African Science: Myth or Reality,* (New York: Vantage Press, 1977), p.12.

70. O.U. Kalu, "Religion, Medicine and Healing in Nigeria". A Keynote Review at the Third Annual Workshop on Medicinal Plants, University of Ife, Ile-Ife, (n.d.) *Op. cit.*, p. 6f.

71. C.C. Achebe, *The World of the Ogbanje,* (Enugu: Fourth Dimension, 1986), *Op. cit.* p.10.

72. I. E. Harrison, "Traditional Healer as a Source of Traditional and Contemporary Powers". in *African Therapeutic Systems,* p.95.

73. B. Oliver, *Medicinal plants in Nigeria.* (Ibadan: The Nigeria College of Arts, Science and Technology, 1960), p.1.

74. P.A. Dopamu, "The Place of *Onisegun* in the Yoruba Health Care System" in *The*

Place of Religion in the Development of Nigeria (ed. by I.A.B. Balogun, P.A. Dopamu et. al. (Ilorin: Dept. of Religion, Unilorin, 1988), p.6

75.   E. I. Metuh, *African Religions in Western Conceptual Schemes, Op. cit.,* p.162.

76.   S. N. Ezeanya, "Healing in Traditional African Society" in *WAR,* Vol. 17, No.1 (1978), p. 6.

77.   E. I. Metuh, *African Religions in Western Conceptual Schemes, Op. cit.,* p.162.

78.   E. Ilogu, *Christianity and Igbo Culture,* (London NOK Publishers, 1974), p.54.

79.   P.A. Talbot, *The Peoples of Southern Nigeria,* Vol. II, (London: Frank Case, 1969), p.187.

80.   A.C. Campbell, "Some Notes on Ngwaketse Divination" in *African Therapeutic Systems, p.56.*

81.   E.G. Parrinder, *West African Religions,* (London: Epworth Press, 1969), p. 137.

82.   S.U. Erivwo, "Epha: Divination System among the Urhobo of Niger Delta" in
  •   *African Notes,* Vol. 8, No. 1, (1979), p. 21.

83.   J.S. Mbiti, *African Religions and Philosophy, Op. cit.,* p. 177.

84.   E. Isichei, *Igbo Worlds: An Anthology of Oral History and Historical Descriptions,* (Philadelphia: Institute of the Study of Human Issues, 1978), p. 172.

85.   F. A. Arinze, *Sacrifice in Ibo Religion,* (Ibadan: Ibadan University Press, 1970), p.64.

86.   E. I. Metuh, *African Religions in Western Conceptual Schemes, Op. cit.,* p.162.

87.   D. Westernmann, *The African Today and Tomorrow.*

88.   Una Maclean, *Magical Medicine: A Nigerian case study, Op. cit.,* p.176.

89.   R. Prince, "Some Notes on Yoruba Native Doctors and their Management of Mental Illness" in Conference Report, First Pan-African Psychiatric Conference, Abeokuta, Nigeria, p. 70.

90.   J.O. Mume, *Traditional Medicine in Nigeria,* (Agbarho: JOM Native Cure Centre, (n.d.) p.1.

91.   J.A.A. Ayoade, "The Concept of Inner Essence in Yoruba Traditional Medicine", *Op. cit.,* p.53.

92.   E.B. Idowu, *African Traditional Religion: A Definition,* (London: S.C.M., 1973), p. 200f.

93.   A.C. Campbell, "Some Notes on Nwaketse Divination" in *African Therapeutic Systems,* p. 56.

94.   F. Nadel, *Nupe Religion,* (London: Routledge and Kegan Paul, 1954).

95.   M.M. Green, *Igbo Village Affairs,* (London: Frank Cass, 2nd edition, 1964).

96.   J.S. Mbiti: *African Religions and Philosophy,* (London: Heinemann, 1969), *Op. cit.*

97.   .... *Introduction to African Religion* (London: Heinemann, 1969).

98.   E.E. Evan-Pritchard, *Witchcraft, Oracle and Magic among the Azande,* (Oxford: Clarendon Press, 1976).

99.   K.A. Opoku, *West African Traditional Religion,* (Accra: F.E.P. International, 1978).

Chapter Two pp: 20-53

1.   A. Afigbo, *Ropes of Sand: Studies in Igbo History and Culture,* (Oxford: O.U.P., 1981), P.3.

2.   C.I. Ejizu, *Ofo: Igbo Ritual Symbol;* (Enugu: Fourth Dimension Publisher, 1986), p.13.

3.   E.I. Metuh, *African Religions in Western Conceptual Schemes,* (Ibadan: Pastoral Institute, 1985), p. 37f.

4.   O.U. Kalu, "Precarious Vision: The African Perception of His World" in *Readings in African Humanities: African Cultural Development,* (ed by). O.U. Kalu (Enugu: Fourth Dimension, 1978), p. 38f.

5.   C.C. Achebe, *The World of the Ogbanje* (Enugu: Fourth Dimension, 1986), p. 10.

6.   A.O.E. Animalu: *Science, Religion and African Culture,* p.8.

7.   V.C. Uchendu: *The Igbo of South East Nigeria,* (New York: Holt, Rinework and Winston, 1985), p.1.

8.   S.O.K. Ezea, "The Pre-Christian Belief in and Cult of the Supreme Being in Anambra and Imo States of Nigeria" *Unpublished M.A. Thesis,* Department of Religion, University of Nigeria, Nsukka 1979, p.3. Some information on Urhobo Cosmology were gleaned from J.O. Ubrurhe, "A Functional Approach to the Study of Taboos: A Case Study of Urhobo Traditional Society" *Unpublished M.A. Project,* Dept. of Religion, University of Nigeria, Nsukka, 1986 pp 10-33.3.

9.   R.E. Bradbury, *The Benin Kingdom and the Edo-Speaking Peoples of South-Western Nigeria,* (London: Whiteman Mountain, 1970), p.14.

10.   J.O. Awolalu and P.A. Dopamu, *West African Traditional Religion,* (Ibadan: Onibonoje press, 1979), p.14.

11.   A.O. Erhueh, *Image of God in Man, (Rome:* Urbaniana University Press, 1987), p. 272.

12.   G.O. Ehusani, *An Afro-Christian Vision,* (Ibadan: The Ambassador Publication, 1972), p. 205.

13.   S.U Erivwo, "Traditional Religion and Christianity among the Urhobo" in E. I. Metuh (ed.) *The Gods in Retreat; Continuity and Change in African Religions,* (Enugu: Fourth Dimension, 1985), p. 22.

14.   *Ibid,* p.22

15.   *Ibid.*

16.   P.A. Talbot, The *Peoples of Southern Nigeria,* Vol. II (London: O.U.P 1926), p.19.

17.   S. N. Ezeanya (Rt. Rev.) "God, Spirit and the Spirit World" in *Biblical Revelation and African Belief,* (Kwesi Dickson *et. al.* (ed.) (London: Lutherwork, 1972), p. 35f.

18.   S. U. Erivwo, *Traditional Religion and Christianity in Nigeria: The Urhobo People,* (Ekpoma: Dept. of Religious Studies and Philosophy, 1991), p.39.

19.   E. I. Ifesieh, (Rev. Fr.) The Concept of Chineke as Reflected in Igbo Names and Proverbs in *Communio Viatorum,* No. XXVI, 1983, p.115.

20.   M. Y. Nabofa, "Survey of Urhobo Traditional Religion" *in The Urhobo People,* O. Otite (ed.) (Ibadan: Heinemann, 1982), pp. 220-223.

21.   S. U. Erivwo, *Traditional Religion and Christianity in Nigeria: The Urhobo People,* Op. cit., pp. 17-18.

22.   Ibid. p. 20.

23.   E. G. Parrinder, *West African Religion,* (London: Epworth, Press, 1961), p. 15.

24.   Interview with Mr. F. Ekama on 24th September, 1985, age 58.

25.   Interview with Mr. S. Aboyehokevwe, 29th September, 1985, age 65.

26.   M. Y. Nabofa, "A Survey of Urhobo Traditional Religion" in *The Urhobo People*, *Op. cit.*, p. 223. Nabofa categorized Urhobo Divinities into four viz: the war, prosperity and fertility, guardian and ethnical divinities: These are the main departments of life. The implication of this categorization is the subtle way of saying that in every aspect of the Urhobo life, there is a divinity. I have discussed their function in the maintenance of the morality, unity and the stability of the traditional Urhobo society. See "Functional Approach to the Study of Taboos: A Case Study of Urhobo Traditional Society." Unpublished M. A. Project, Department of Religion, University of Nigeria, Nsukka, 1986, pp. 15-22.

27.   R. E. Bradbury; *The Benin Kingdom and Edo-Speaking Peoples of South-Western Nigeria* (London: Wightman Mountain, 1970), p. 160f.

28.   M. O. Adasu, *Understanding African Traditional Religion;* Part One (Sherborne: Dorset Publishing Co. 1985), p. 19f.

29.   J. S. Mbiti, *African Religions and Philosophy*, Op, Cit., p. 33.

30.   S. U. Erivwo; *Traditional Religion and Christianity in Nigeria: The Urhobo People*, *Op. cit.*, p. 25.

31.   J. S. Mbiti, *African Religions and Philosophy*, Op, cit., p. 33.

32.   R. E. Bradbury, *The Benin Kingdom and Edo-Speaking Peoples of South-Western Nigeria*, p. 160. I have discussed the cult of the ancestor in details. See "Functional Approach to the Study of Taboos: A Case Study of Urhobo Traditional Society", *Unpublished* M.A. Project, U.N. Nsukka, 1986, pp. 22-27.

33.   S. U. Erivwo: "Religion and Identity: The Church's Role in Nation Building with Special Reference to Nigeria" in *NASR*, 1988, p. 3.

34.   Sulayman Nyany: *Islam, Christianity and Africa* (Vermont: 1984), p.21.

35.   C. I. Ejizu, "Healing as Wholeness: The Igbo Experience" *Africana Marburhensia*, Vol. 20, NO. 1, 1987, p. 13. The Akans conceive man as more exalted than the deities hence they believe that the deities exist for the interest of man and could be censured by man. Gyekye puts it that "if they (deities) deliver the goods, they are worshipped and adored, if they fail, they are viewed with contempt, (see Kwame Gyekye, *An Essay on African Philosophical Thought*, (New York; Cambridge University Press, 1987) p.137. Many Africans or foreign writers on African religion, history, anthropology, literature especially culture have at one time or the other asserted that African tradition emphasizes community, family and progeny, and that the maintenance of wholesome human relations and hospitality are essential marks of the traditional African. (K. A. Busia, *The Challenge of Africa*, (New York: Frederick A. Praegar, 1962),

Kenneth Kaunda, *A Humanist in Africa,* (Nashbille: Abingbon Press, 1966), John Mbiti, *African Religions and Philosophy,* (London: Heinemann, 1970), W.E.B. Dubois, *The Souls of Blackfolk,* (Greanwich Co. Faweett, 1961), Dubois, *The World and Africa,* (Cambridge and Massachusetts: Harvard University Press, 1962) Simeon and Phoebe Ottenberg (eds.) *Cultures and Societies in Africa,* (New York: Random Press, 1960), Julius Nyerere, "Ujaama — The Basis of African Socialism" *in African Socialism,* (ed. by William Friedland and Carl Rosberg), (Standard: Stanford University Press, 1967. W. E. Abraham, *The Mind of Africa,* (Chicago: The University of Chicago Press, 1962); Chieka Ifemesia, *Traditional Humane Living Among the Igbo: An Historical Perspective,* (Enugu: Fourth Dimension, 1979).

36.   G.O. Ehusani, *An Afro-Christian Vision "Ozovehe",* (Ibadan: Ambassador, 1992), p.2. Benezet Bujo affirms the African attachment of much importance to life. (Lee Peter Schineller, *A Handbook on Inculturation* (New York: Paulist Press, 1990), p.79. An American Missionary notes the different manifestations and forms of the Nigerian wonderful respect and love of life. He asserts that although this concept may sound vague and general, that in Nigeria "One lives close to life; one lives close to death, and hence gains a deeper appreciation for life." (Lee Darmain Mussanda, "Life as a Gift and Task" in African Christian Studies, (Nairobi, July 1986), p.87. However, Ehusani succinctly argues that "Life and its promotion and protection is the central pre-occupation of the African family, clan, chiefdom, whose legal and authority structures have in turn been designed to foster life". Human actions are good or bad to the extent that they promote or threaten life. (G.O. Ehusani) *An Afro-Christian Vision, Ozovehe,* 1992, p. 210).

37.   P. Tempel, *Bantu Philosophy,* (Paris: Presence Africaine, 1959), p.78.

38.   R.S. Rattray, *Religion and Art in Ashanti,* p. 163.

39.   E.I. Metuh, *Comparative Studies of African Traditional Religions,* p.25. Metuh quoted A.G. Leonard, *Lower Niger and Its Tribes,* (London: 1966), p. 429.

40.   O.U. Kalu, An Alive Universe: The African World Over a Century's Presence of the Church in Africa: A Historical Analysis of the Evangelization Process, p.1.

41.   J.S. Mbiti, *African Religions and Philosophy, Op. cit.,* p.16.

42.   O.U. Kalu, "Precarious Vision: The African Perception of His World" in *Reading in African Humanities: African Culture Development, Op. cit.,* P.39.

:3.   J.S. Mbiti, *African Religions and Philosophy, Op. cit.,* p.17.

44. Kwame Gyekye, *An Essay on African Philosophical Thought* ; (New York: Cambridge University Press, 1987), p.70.

45. S. Nyang, *Islam, Christianity and African Identity,* (Vermont, 1984), p.20.

46. *Ibid.,* p.22. See Ehusani, G.O. : *An Afro-Christian Vision,* p. 88.

47. J.F. Smurl, *Religious Ethics, A System Approach* (New Jersey: Prentice Hall, 1972), p.38.

48. Wole Soyinka, *Idanre and Other Poems;* (London: Eyre Methuen, 1967), p. 65.

49. O.U. Kalu, "Precarious Vision: African Perception of His World" in *Reading in African Humanities, Op. cit.,* p.40.

50. J.O. Ubrurhe, "Man and the Concept of Hereafter in African Belief System" in AJRS (Abraka Journal of Religious Studies), Vol.1, No. 1, July (1991), p.7.

51. O.U. Kalu, "Precarious Vision: African Perception of His World" in *Reading in Humanities, Op. cit.,* p.40.

52. C. Ifemesia, *Issues in African Studies and National Education,* Selected Works of Kenneth Onwuka Dike (Kenneth Onwuka Dike Centre (KODIC), Awka, 1978), p. 38. Quoted by A. O. Animalu, "Science, Religion and African Culture", p. 3.

53. A. O. Animalu, "Science, Religion and African Culture" Being a Lecture Delivered in a Seminar Organized by the Academy of Science at the Nigerian Institute of International Affairs, Victoria Island, Lagos on 8th April, 1989, p.1.

54. *Ibid.,* p. 8.

55. I. G. Pawson, *Physical Anthropology: Human Evolution, (New* York: John Wiley and Sons, 1977), pp. 124 & 125.

56. Interview with Pa Iyoya on 4th April, 1992, p. 110

57. M. Y. Nabofa, "Erhi and Eschatology" in *Traditional Religion in West Africa,* (ed.), E. A. Adegbola (Ibadan: Daystar, 1983), p. 298.

58. J. O. Awolalu, *Yoruba Belief and Sacrificial Rites,* (London: Longman, 1981), pp. 13 & 33. Also see E. B. Idowu: Olodumare: *God in Yoruba Belief,* p.169f.

59. G. E. Okeke, "The Interpretation of New Testament Teaching on Death and Future life in an African Context" *Unpublished Ph.D. Thesis,* Dept. of Religion, U.N.N. (1981), p.10.

60. R. Horton, "African Traditional Thought and Western Science" in *AFRICA, Vol.* 37, Nos 1-2, January and April, (1967) p.55.

61. M. M. Iwu, "Symbolism and Selectivity in Traditional African Medicine" A Lecture Delivered by the Winner of the Vice-Chancellor's Research Leadership Prize for 1987, University of Nigeria, Nsukka, January 12, (1989), p. 3.

62. N. S. Booth (Jr.), "An Approach to African Religion" in *African Religions: A Symposium*, p. 6. Also see J. S. Mbiti, *African Religions and Philosophy*, p. 92, Mbiti's concept of Africa worldview as anthropocentric is explicated thus: African people considered man to be at the centre of the universe. He sees the universe in terms of himself and endeavours to live in harmony with it. Even where there is no biological life in an object, African people attribute (mystical) life to it, in order to establish a more direct relationship with the world around them. In this way, the visible and invisible parts of the universe are at man's disposal through physical, mystical and religious means, p. 89 (John Mbiti, *Introduction to African Religions and Philosophy*, (London: Heinemann, 1975) p. 39, See Dominique Zahan; *The Religion, Spirituality and Thought of Traditional Africa* (Translated by Kato Ezra and Lawrence Martin, Chicago: Chicago University Press, 1979), p. 61.

63. E. I. Metuh, *African Religions in Western Conceptional Scheme: The Problem of Interpretation, Op. cit.*, p. 162.

64. U. Maclean, *Magical Medicine: A Nigerian Case Study*, (London: Reading and Fakahnam, 1971), p. 28. Dopamu also argues that to allow a divinity to give vent to his indignation, to fail in one's loyalty to a divinity, to make a breach of cultic interdiction, is to aid the trammels of man's total well-being.

65. W. Z. Conco, "The African Bantu Traditional Practice of Medicine: Some Preliminary Observations" in *African Therapeutic systems* (ed.) by Z. A. Ademuwagun, et. al. (Massachusetts: Crossroads Press, 1979), p. 58.

66. O. U. Kalu: "Precarious Vision: The African Perception of His World" in *Reading in African Humanities, Op. cit.*, p. 38f.

67. Genesis 1 : 26-31.

68. J. O. Ubrurhe; Functional Approach to the Study of Taboos: A Case Study of Urhobo Traditional Society" *Unpublished M. A. Thesis, Dept. of Religion, University of Nigeria, Nsukka (1986), p.98.*

69. *Genesis* 1: 28-29.

70. J.A.A. Ayoade, "The Concept of Inner Essence in Yoruba Traditional Medicine" in African *Therapeutic Systems*, (ed) by, Z. A. Ademuwagun et. al. (Massachussets: Crossroads Press, 1979), p. 50.

71. G.W. Harley, *Native African Medicine with Special Reference to Its Practice in the Mano Tribe of Liberia*, (London: Frank Case, 1970), p.37.

72. A. Smith of Cyprus, *A Contribution to South African Materia Medica*, (Lovedale: South Africa, 1988), p.5.

73. A. Alland (Jr.) *Adaptation in Cultural Evolution: An approach to medical anthropology*, (New York: Columbia Uni/ersity Press, 1970), p. 127.

74. D.C. Sills, International Encyclopaedia of Social Sciences Vol. 5 & 6: (New York: Macmillan and Free Press, 1972), p.330.

75. L. Hirvonen, "Healing, Culture and the Concept of Human" in *Journal of Mission Theology*, Vol.1, Fasc. 1, (1991), p.94. Also see F. Brockington, *World Health*, (Harmondsworth, Middlesex: Penguin Books, 1958).

76. *Ibid.*, p.94.

77. *Ibid.*, p.94.

78. J.O. Mume, *A Message for All Who Seek Health. (Agbarho:* Jom Tradomedical Naturopathic Hospital, 1973), p.3.

79. J.O. Mume, *Traditional Medicine in Nigeria*, (Agbarho Jom Nature Cure Centre, n.d.), p.41.

80. W.S. Mensah-Dapa, "Observation on Traditional Healing Methods in Ghana" in *African Therapeutic Systems*, (ed.) by Z.A. Ademuwagun et.al. (Massachusetts: Crossroad, 1979), p.113.

81. J. Aagaard. "The Cosmology Behind Healing Techniques" in *Journal of Mission Theology*, Vol.1. Fasc. 1 (1991), p.6.

82. Z.A. Ademuwagun, "Problem and Prospect of Legitimatizing and Integrating Aspect of Traditional Health Care Systems and Methods with Modern Medical Therapy" in *African Therapeutic Systems, p.* 160.

83. I. Hirvonen, "Healing, Culture and the Concept of Human" in *Journal of Mission Theology*, p.97. Also see L. Payer, *Medicine and Culture*, (New York; Penguin Books, 1988).

84. A.B.T. Byaruhanga-Akiiki, The Theology of Medicine in *Journal of African Religion*, Vol.2, No. 1, (1991), p. 26.

85. P.A. Dopamu, "Yoruba Magic and Medicine and Their Relevance for Today" in *Religions NARS*, Vol.4, Dec. (1991), p. 12.

86. J.A.A. Ayoade, "The Concept of Inner Essence in Yoruba Traditional Medicine"

in *African Therapeutic Systems,* (ed.) by Z.A. Ademuwagun *et.al.* (Massachusetts: Crossroads Press, (1979), p. 49.

87.   E.G. Parrinder, *African Traditional Religion,* (London: Sheldon Press, Third Edition, 1974), p.126f.

88.   W.Z. Conco, "The African Bantu Traditional Practices of Medicine: Some Preliminary Observation in *African Therapeutic Systems",* (ed. by), Z.A. Ademuwagun *et.al.* Op. cit., p.62.

89.   Interview with Ovie of Oghara, 1985. See J.O. Ubrurhe, "A Functional Approach to the Study of Taboos", pp.82-90.

90.   M. Gelfand, *Medicine and Custom in Africa* (Edinburgh and London: E. & S. Livingstone 1964), p. VI.

91.   W.Z. Conco, "The African Bantu Traditional Practice of Medicine. Some Preliminary Observation" in *African Therapeutic Systems,* p.58.

92.   M. Gelfand, *Medicine and Custom in Africa,* p. 38.

93.   J.O. Mume, *Tradomedicalism: What it is?* (Agbarho: JOM Nature Cure Centre, n.d.), p.49.

94.   G.Bibeau, E. Corin *et. al., Traditional Medicine in Zaire: Present and Potential contribution to the Health Series,* (International Development Research Centre, 1980), p.17.

95.   J.O. Mume, *Traditional Medicine in Nigeria,* p. 65. Mume also discusses the eight therapeutic methods and this information is gleaned from his work.

96.   A.J. Youngson, *The Scientific Revolution in Victorian Medicine,* (New York: Homes and Meier Publisher, 1979), p.6.

97.   *Ibid.,* p.70.

98.   J.O. Mume, *Traditional Medicine in Nigeria, Op. cit.,* p.71

99.   N. Ezeabasili, *African Science: Myth or Reality* (New York: Vantage Press, 1977), p.53.

100.   E.O. Okolugbo, "The Olise-Igbe Religious Movement" in *Socio Philosophical Perspective of African Traditional Religion* (eds.), E. Ekpunobi & I. Ezeaku (Enugu: New Age Publisher, 1990), p. 24. E.O. Okolugbo has described the hierarchy in its priesthood and their function. From the exchange of letters between Bernard Uyo, Omonedo's son and the ADO of Ase District when Omonode was arrested and subsequently convicted, the elucidation of the main issues involved in this aspect of Urhobo Traditional Religion was aided.

101. F. Fanon, *The Wretched of the Earth,* (France: Francois Maspero editeur, 1961), p. 32.

102. J.V. Taylor, *The Prime Vision,* (London: S.C.M. 1969), p.67.

103. E. Amadi, *The Concubine,* (Ibadan: Heinemann, Reprinted 1988), pp. 157-9.

104. The interesting thing about this medicine was that the author was discussing with a friend who had problem in securing a job. He was disappointed in all the interviews he attended until he consulted a diviner who told him that evil forces were responsible for his disappointments in all the interviews he attended. The diviner advised him to use the medicine before attending another interview which he did and succeeded. The author advised a friend who found it difficult to get a girl to marry. We attributed his problem to the evil machinations of one of the girls he disappointed. After the performance of the medicine, a girl who nearly abandoned him later changed her mind. Today they are happy couple.

105. J. Munonye, *Obi* (London: Heinemann, 1976), p. 110.

106. Interview with Mr. J.U. Edakarabor on 23rd January, 1992, Age 50.

107. S.N. Ezeanya, "Healing in African Traditional Society" in *WAR,* Vol.17, No. 1, (1978).

108. J. Munonye, *Obi* p.158.

109. Isidore Okpewho, *The Victim,* (Ikeja : Longman Drumboat, 1979), pp.180-97.

110. J. Munonye, *Obi* pp.115-6.

111. M.Gelfand, *The African Witch* (Edinburgh, London, E.S. Livingstone, 1967), p.137.

112. Interview with Chief Atuya of Okpara Waterside on 2nd October, 1985, Age 58. See J.O. Ubrurhe, "A Functional Approach to the study of Taboos: A Case Study of Urhobo Traditional Society", p. 89.

113. P.A. Dopamu, "The Forces of Evil and their Social Functions Among the Yoruba" *NASR,* No. 1. September 1979), p. 39. He also argues that in Africa, people still believe in the evil machinations of sorcerers and witches. It is generally believed that these people are evilly disposed and anti-social and they disrupt the well-being of individual as well as the society, by causing misfortune, illness, poverty, barrenness, ill-luck, death and other evils.

P.A. Dopamu, "The Secret of Total-Well-Being with Particular Reference to African Religion" in *JARS* (Journal of Arabic and Religious Studies), Vol.1, Dec. (1984), p.7.

114.   J.S. Mbiti, *African Religions and Philosophy, Op. cit., p.* 202.

115.   E.G. Parrinder, *African Traditional Religion, Op. cit.* p. 123.

116.   V. Omuabor, "Face to Face with Juju Man" in *African Concord,* Vol. 38, April, (1987), p.14.

117.   P. Esiri, "Witchcraft in Urhobo" *Unpublished B.A. (Ed.) Project Work,* Dept. of Religious Studies, Bendel State University, Abraka Campus, June (1988), p.14. Also see Fortes and Dieter (ed.) *African Systems of Thought* (Norwich: O.U.P., 1972) and E. Evans Pritchard, *Witchcraft, Oracle and Magic Among the Azande,* is very informative and relevant for the discussion on witchcraft. For instance, Forte and Dieter have 205 case files on witchcraft activities in Africa.

Chapter Three pp: 54-101

1.   Interview with Ishanive of Arhavwarien on 7th August, 1991, Aged 80.

2.   Interview with Mr. Odiru Onorohwovo of Ebo-Orogun on 29th November, 1991, Aged 75.

3.   Interview with Chief D.O. Adasin on 20th November, 1991, Aged 56.

4.   Interview with Mrs. Onosemuode on 23rd November, 1991, Aged 35.

5.   Interview with Dr B.J.E. Itsueli, Delta State University, Abraka on 6th September, 1992.

6.   A.C. Campbell, "Some Notes on Ngwaketse Divination" in *African Therapeutic Systems,* (ed.) by Z.A. Ademuwagun, *et. al.* (Massachusett: Crossroad Press, 1979), p. 57.

7.   S.U.Erivwo, "Epha: Divination System among the Urhobo of Niger Delta" in *African Notes,* Vol. 8, No.1 (1979), p. 22.

8.   Z.A. Ademuwagun, "Problem of and Prospect of Legitimatizing and Integrating Aspects of Traditional Health Care Systems and Methods with Modern Medical Therapy" in *African Therapeutic Systems,* p. 161.

9.   *Ibid.,* p.161.

10.   J.O. Mume, *Tradomedicalism: What it is,* (Agbarho: JOM Nature Cure Centre n.d.), p. 43.

11.   U. Maclean, Magical *Medicine: A Nigerian case study,* (London: Reading and Fakennam, 1971, p. 21f.

12. P. Tempel, *Bantu Philosophy,* (Paris: Presence Africaine, 1959), p.78.

13. J. Jahn, *Muntu: An outline of the New African Culture,* (New York: Grove Press, 1961), p.100 - See J.S. Mbiti, *African Religions and Philosophy* (London: Heinemann, 1969), p.11.

14. J. Mouroux, *The Meaning of Man,* (New York: Sheed and Ward, 1948), p. 128.

15. *Ibid.,* p. 133; See A.U. Uzoma, "The Causal Role of the Word" (Okwu) in Igbo Traditional Medicine: A Paper Presented at the Third Annual Seminar in Igbo Life and Culture organized by the Institute of African Studies in Association with the Faculty of Arts, U.N. Nsukka, December 3-6, 1989, p.10.

16. L.D. Reemaeker, *The Philosophy of Being: A Synthesis of Metaphysics,* (London: Herder Book, 1966), p. 274. See A.U. Uzoma, *Ibid,* p.10.

17. M.M. Iwu, "Symbolism and Selectivity in Traditional African Medicine". A Lecture Delivered by the Winner of Vice-Chancellor's Research Leadership Prize for 1987, U.N. Nsukka, January 12, 1989, p.3.

18. E.B. Idowu, *African Traditional Religion: A Definition* (London: S.C.M. 1973), p.201.

19. M.M. Iwu, "Symbolism and Selectivity in Traditional African Medicine", *Op. cit.,* p. 10.

20. J. Jahn, *Muntu: An outline of the new African culture, Op. cit.,* p.134.

21. J.S. Mbiti, *African Religions and Philosophy,* (London: Heinemann, 1969), p. 167.

22. J.O. Kokwora, *Medical Plant in East African ,* (Nairobi: East African Literature Bureau, 1976), p.4.

23. Madam Oti is a medicine woman in Okurekpo. She handles cases of Natural, Preternatural and Supernatural diseases. Interviewed on 2nd February, 1992, Aged 60.

24. J.O. Awolalu and P.A. Dopamu, *West African Traditional Religion,* (Ibadan: Onibonoje Press, 1979), p.146.

25. J.S. Mbiti; *African Religion and Philosophy, Op. cit.,* p.166.

26. U. Maclean, *Magical Medicine: A Nigerian case study, Op. cit.,* p. 76.

27. R. Prince, "Some Notes on Yoruba Native Doctors and their Management of Mental Illness" in Conference Report, First Pan-African Psychiatric Conference, Abeokuta, Nigeria, p. 70.

28.   Interview with Madam Oti of Okurekpo on 2nd February, 1992, Aged 65.

29.   J.O. Mume, *Traditional Medicine in Nigeria,* (Agbarho: JOM Nature Cure Centre (n.d.), p.1.

30.   Interview with Mr. E. Okpukoro on 10th March, 1992, Aged 45, He told a story of how a palm branch, pricked and stuck in his father's (a palm collector) leg. All efforts to remove it was to no avail. The leg became swollen and septic to the extent that they were despondent. One night, in a dream, his grandfather who had died showed his father the medicine to remove the thorn. That in the same night, his grandfather in a dream showed his mother the same medicine emphasizing that he (grandfather) knew that his son was forgetful. When the medicine was applied on the leg, the thorn came out on its own.

31.   M.J. Field, *Religion and Medicine of Ga People,* (London: Oxford University · Press. Reprinted 1961), p. 114.

32.   E.G. Parrinder, *West African Religion,* London: Geoffrey Chapman, 1949), p.157.

33.   A.U. Uzoma, "The Causal Role of the Word" (Okwu) in Igbo Traditional Medicine". A Paper Presented at the Third Annual Seminar in "Igbo Life and Culture" organized by the Institute of African Studies in Association with the Faculty of Arts, U.N. Nsukka, December 3-6, 1989, p.10.

34.   E.G. Parrinder, *West African Religion Op. cit., p.152*

35.   E.I. Metuh, *African Religions in Western Conceptual Schemes,* (Ibadan: Pastoral Institute, 1985), p. 112.

36.   *Ibid.,* p. 163.

37.   S.N. Ezeanya, "Healing in Traditional African Society" in *WAR,* Vol. 17. No.1, (1978), p.6.

38.   Interview with Mr. F. Ekama on 17/10/91. This sacrifice was performed by the head of the family because the offence was committed against the ancestors. If he had committed the offence against a divinity, the priest of the divinity would have performed the ritual. Mr. Ekama explained that the elders of the family accepted and participated in the sacrifice with much reluctance. For in grievous offences like this, the offender is usually left to suffer and die. The goat, the sacrificial victim, dies a vicarious death in order to save the life of the offender.

39.   D.R. Harjula; "The Human Struggle with Guilt" in *Journal of Mission Theology,* Vol.1, Fasc 1, (1991), p.31.

40.   S.U. Erivwo, "Epha: Divination System Among the Urhobo of Niger Delta" in *African Notes* Vol. 8, No.1 (1979), p. 21.

41. *Ibid.*, p.21f.

42. A Shorter; *African Culture and the Christian Church*, (London: Geoffrey Chapman, 1973), p. 136

43. U. Maclean, *Magical Medicine: A Nigerian case study, Op. cit.*, p. 30.

44. R. Horton, "African Traditional Thought and Western Science" in *AFRICA*, Vol. 37, Nos. 1-2, January and April, (1967), p. 55.

45. J. Mok. Goodchild, "Biblical Theology and the Healing Ministry" in *WAR* Vol. 17, No.1, (1976), p.27.

46. *Ibid.*, p. 47.

47. A.O. Iwuagwu (Rt. Rev.) "The Healing Ministry in the Church in Nigeria" in *WAR*, Vol.17, No.1, (1978), p.47

48. *Ibid.*, p.46

49. S.N. Ezeanya, (Rt. Rev.) "Healing in Traditional African Society" in *WAR*, Vol. 17. No.1, (1978), p.15.

50. U. Maclean, *Magical Medicine: A Nigerian Case Study, Op. cit.*, p. 156.

51. N. Ezeabasili, *African Science: Myth or Reality*, (New York: Vantage Press, 1977), p. 12.

52. U. Maclean, *Magical Medicine: A Nigerian Case Study, Op. cit.*, p. 30.

53. World Health Organization (1975), Quoted by Oyebola, D.D.O. National Medical Policies in Nigeria in *Professionalization of African Medicine*, (ed.) by Last, M. and Chavunduka, G.E. Manchester: Manchester University Press, 1986), p.221.

54. M. Mead, *Culture, Health and Disease*, (London: Tavistock Publication Limited, 1966), p.21.

55. C. Nze, "Logic in African Charm Medicine" in *Nigerian Journal of Social Studies*, *Vol.4*, No.1, (1987), p.31.

56. *Ibid.*, p. 31.

57. J. Gorju, "Ethnography of the English part of the Victoria of Uganda" see D. Zeller, Basawo Baganda: "The Traditional Doctor of Buganda" in *African Therapeutic Systems*, (ed.) by Z.A. Ademuwagun *et. al.* (Massachusetts: Crossroad Press, 1979), p. 141.

58.   Research in Native Medicine in Daily Times, September 25, (1975), p.8.

59.   A.E. Ohiaeri (n.d.), A Research in the Traditional Nigerian Medicine, Medical Centre, University of Nigeria, Nsukka, p.6.

60.   M. Gelfand, *Medicine and Custom in Africa* (Edinburgh and London: E. & S. Livingstone 1964), p. 4.

61.   "Traditional Medicine and National Development" in National Concord Monday, February 9, (1987), p.9.

62.   P.A. Dopamu, "The Place of Onisegun in the Yoruba Health Care System" in *The Place of Religion in the Development of Nigeria* (ed.) by I.A.B. Balogun, P.A. Dopamu et. al. (Ilorin: Dept. of Religion, Unilorin, 1988), p. 20f. See *Sunday Sketch*, Feb. 2. (1986), p.6. Also see T. Hockmayer, "Traditional Medicine Revisited" in *Daily Times*, August 12, (1975), p.7.

63.   C. Nze, "Logic in African Charm Medicine" in *The Nigerian Journal of Social Studies,* Vol. 4, No.1, Oct., 1987, p.25. U.S. Anderson also argues that man is the essence of the mighty intelligence, which guides and controls the universe. That man not only lives in this intelligence but also part of it and the whole of it... This intelligence, he argues, is for man to use as he sees fit. U.S. Anderson, *Three Magic Words* (California: Wilshire Book 1954), p. 8.

64.   P.A. Dopamu, "Health and Healing within the Traditional African Religious Context" in *ORITA*, Vol 17, No. 2, Dec. (1985), p. 74.

65.   V.M. Turner, *The Forest of Symbols,* (London: Connel University Press, 1967), p.19.

66.   A. Shorter, *African Culture and the Christian Church,* (London: Geoffrey Chapman, 1973), p. 122.

67.   M Wilson, "Nyakayusa, Ritual and Symbolism" in *American Anthropologists,* Vol. 56, No. 2, (1954), p. 241.

68.   Encyclopaedia Britannica Vol. 15, p. 863

69.   A.N.O. Ekwunife, "Consecration in Igbo Traditional Religion" *Unpublished Ph.D. Thesis,* Dept. of Religion, University of Nigeria Nsukka. 1986, pp. 33-34.

70.   E.N. Zuesse, *Ritual Cosmos,* (Otuo: Ohio University Press, (1979), p.242.

71.   G. Bibeau, E. Corin et. al. *Traditional Medicine in Zaire, Present and Potential Contribution to the Health Service.* (Ottawa: International Development Centre, 1980), p. 18.

72. Interview with Chief Dr. R.A.O. Uko on 23rd June, 1992, Aged 70, Chief Uko was the National Vice-President of Nigerian Association of Medical Herbalists.

73. *Ibid.*

74. Interview with Simeon Adanumueke 28/6/90, Aged 69.

75. Interview with a woman.

76. J.O. Ubrurhe, "A Functional Approach to the Study of Taboos: A Case Study of Urhobo Traditional Society", *Unpublished M.A. Thesis,* Dept. of Religion, U.N.N., 1986, pp. 88-89.

77. U. Maclean, *Magical Medicine: A Nigerian Case Study* (London: Reading and Fakenham 1971), p.13.

78. J.A.A. Ayoade, "The Concept of Inner Essence in Yoruba Traditional Medicine" in *African Therapeutic Systems,* (ed. by) Z. A. Ademuwagun, et.al. (Massachusetts: Crossroad Press, 1979), p. 49.

79. A. Shorter, *African Culture and the Christian Church, Op. cit.,* p. 131.

80. Mr Odiru Onorohwovo is a renowned traditional osteopathist at Eboh-Orogun. In his treatment of fractures, he usually breaks the leg of a hen. He then uses the remedy to tie both the patient's leg and that of the hen after massaging and arranging the broken bones in their right position. The response of the patient is witnessed from how the hen behaves with the leg. Immediately after the treatment, the hen cannot stand with the leg. It will gradually stand with the broken leg as it responds to the treatment. Mr. Odiru claimed that after treating late Patrick Idjerhe who had an accident and could not be treated at Igbobi and Eku Hospitals, the doctors came to buy the medicine from him, a request which he did not concede to. During the process of treatment, Mr. Odiru massages the affected leg to ensure that the bones are properly held in their position.

81. Interview with Mr. B. Odafe on 27/7/91, Aged 45.

82. J.S. Mbiti, *The Prayers of African Religion,* (London: SPCK, 1975), p.38. Also see E.E. Evans-Pritchard, *Nuer Religion,* (London: U.U.P., 1978), p. 105.

83. Interview with Ven. Archdeacon N.A. Enuku, now Bishop of Warri Diocese.

84. Interview with Madam Ekpetiudi Ubrurhe on 30/7/91, Aged 104.

85. M.M. Iwu, "Symbolism and Selectivity in *African Traditional Medicine*" p.5.

86. P.A. Dopamu, "Health and Healing within the Traditional African Religious Context" in *ORITA,* p. 70.

87.   Jackson in his book, *The Role of Faith in the Process of Healing* (London: S.C.M. Press, 1981) emphasize how faith is essential not only for the life of man but also for his health as man.

88.   "Traditional Medicine and National Development" in *National Concord,* Monday, February 9, 1987, p.9.

89.   Interview with Mr. S.N. Enunuaye, Principal of Eradadjaye Grammar School, Adagbrasa - Ugolo, Okpe.

Chapter Four pp: 102-112

1.   Interview with M. Mafuru, Principal Health Officer and the Coordinator, Primary Health Care, for Okpe Local Government Area on 16th July, 1992.

2.   E.I. Metuh, *African Religions in Western Conceptual Schemes,* (Ibadan: Pastoral Institute, 1985), p. 41.

3.   B. Bujo, "Can Morality Be Christian in Africa?" in *African Christian Studies,* (Nairobi, March, 1988) p. 27. Also see G. O. Ehusani, *Afro-Christian Vision:* (Ibadan: Ambassador Publications, 1992), p.226.

4.   P. Bohannan and P. Curtin, *African and Africans* (Revised edition) (New York: The Nature Natural History Press, 1971), p.117.

5.   E. Ward, "The Yoruba Husband-Wife Code" in *Anthropological Series,* No. 6 (Washington, D.C.: Catholic University of America, 1938), p. 41.

6.   G. M. Foster, "Disease Etiologies in Non-Western Medical Systems" in *American Anthropologist,* No. 78 (1976), pp. 173-82.

7.   Interview with Dr. F. O. Esiri, Director, Esiri Hospital, Warri on 22nd July, 1992.

8.   N. H. Wolff, "Concept of Causation and Treatment in Yoruba Medical System: The Special Case of Barrenness" in *African Therapeutic Systems,* (ed.) by Z. A. Ademuwagun et. al. (Massachusetts: Crossroad Press, 1979),p. 130.

9.   Interview with a fellow lecturer, name withheld for security reason.

10.   R. Prince, "The Yoruba Image of the Witch" in *Journal of Mental Science,* No. 107, (1961), pp. 793-805.

11.   Interview with Mr. Ajuya of Okpariabe on 13/10/92; in the *Guardian* of Thursday 22nd July, 1993, Elizabeth Kafaru, a member of the National Association of Alternative Medicine Practitioners, discussed the pains of impotency and sterility and their herbal remedies. "Herbal Remedies" now forms a column in the *Guardian* of Thursday of every week.

12. W. R. Bascom, "Ifa Divination: Communication between God and Man" in *West Africa,* (Bloomington: Indiana University Press, 1969), p.61. Also see Bascom, *The Yoruba of South-Western Nigeria,* (Holt: Rinehart and Winston, 1969), p.61.

13. S. N. Ezeanya "Healing in Traditional African Society" in *WAR,* Vol. 17, No.1 (1978), p. 12.

14. P.A. Dopamu, "Health and Healing Within the Traditional African Religious Context" in *ORITA,* Vol 17, No2, Dec. (1985), p. 76.

15. "The Place of *Onisegun* in the Yoruba Health Care System" in *The Place of Religion in the Development of Nigeria* (ed.) I.A.B. Balogun, P.A. Dopamu *et. al.* (Ilorin: Dept. of Religions, University of Ilorin, 1988), p. 227.

16. Interview with Mr. D. Ogagan, a bonesetter at Agbarho and Mr. Onorohwovo of Eboh-Orogun.

17. Interview with Mr. Oko of Abraka on 7th Sept., 1992.

18. E. B. Idowu, *African Traditional Religion: A Definition,* (London: S. C. M. 1973).

19. C.I. Ejizu, "Healing as Wholeness: The Igbo Experience" in *Africana Marburgensia.* R.I.J. Hacket (ed.) Vol. 129, (1988), p.15.

20. Interview with Okohwake of Arhavwarien on 25th February, 1991, Aged 80.

21. Interview with J. O. Mume on 9th November, 1991, Mume's view was also corroborated by S.N. Ununuaye in my interview with him.

22. "The Place of *Onisegun* in the Yoruba Health Care System" in *The Place of Religion in the Development of Nigeria, Op. cit.,* p.230

23. U. Maclean, *Magical Medicine: A Nigerian Case Study,* (London: Reading and Fakenham, 1971), p. 75.

24. P.A. Dopamu, "The Place of *Onisegun* in the Yoruba Health Care System" *Op. cit.,* p.227.

25. S. N. Ezeanya "Healing in Traditional African Society" *Op. cit.,* p.14.

26. G. Bibeau, E. Corin *et. al,. Traditional Medicine in Zaire: Present and Potential Contribution to the Health Series.* (International Development Research Centre, 1980), p. 14.

27. *Ibid.,* p. 18.

28. Abayomi Sofowora, *Medicinal Plants and Traditional Medicine in Africa,* (Ibadan: Spectrum Books Ltd., 1984), p. 104.

29.   Interview with Okpako of Okparabe on 16th August, 1991, Aged 68.

30.   Interview with Onohwakpo Umukoro of Adeje, 20th August, 1991.

31.   J. U. Oguakwa "Authenticity of African Traditional Medicine Validity and Provocative Consequence: A New Philosophical Dimension in Traditional Medicine" being a Paper Presented at the International Workshop on "African Philosophy in a Scientific and Technological Age", University of Nigeria, Nsukka, June 13-16, 1990, p. 4.

32.   R. I. Arubalueze, "Traditional Medicine in Igbo Society: Critical Issues" in *Socio-Philosophical Perspective of African Traditional Religion,* (ed. by) E. Ekpunobi and I. Ezeaku (Enugu: New Age Publishers, 1990), p.9.

33.   M.M. Iwu. *Traditional Igbo Medicine,* Report of a Project Sponsored by the Institute of African Studies, University of Nigeria, Nsukka, (1981), p. 9.

34.   A.J. Youngson, *The Scientific Revolution in Victorian Medicine,* (New York: Holmes and Meter Publishers, 1979), p.38.

35.   *Ibid.,* p.160.

Chapter Five pp: 113-117

1.   L. R Schwartz, "The Hierarchy of Resort in Curative Practice: The Admirality Islands, Malanesia" in *Journal of Health and Social Behaviour,* No. 10 (1969) pp.201-219.

2.   U. Maclean, *Magical Medicines: A Nigerian Case Study,* (London: Allan Lane, 1971).

3.   J.M Janzen, "Pluralistic Legitimation of Therapeutic Systems in Contemporary Zaire" in *Traditional Healers: Use and Non-use in Health Care Delivery,* I. E. Harrison and D. W. Dunlop (eds.) (Michigan: Michigan State University, 1974), pp. 105-22.

4.   I. Press "Urban Illness: Physicians, Cures and Dual Use in Bogata" in *Journal of Health and Social Behaviour,* No. 10 (1969) pp. 108-18

5.   P.A Twumasi, "Scientific Medicine: The Ghanaian Experience" in *International Journal of Nursing,* No. 9 (1972) pp. 63-75.

6.   I.E Harrison, "Healers as a Source of Traditional and Contemporary Power" in *African Therapeutic Systems,* (ed. by) Z. A. Ademuwagun by *et. al.* (Massachusetts: Crossroads Press, 1979), p. 97.

7.   W. Rodney, *How Europe Underdeveloped Africa* (Dar Es Salam: Tanzania, 1972), pp. 264-73.

8.   P. Fanon, *The Wretched of the Earth,* (New York: Penguin Books, 1977 Reprinted), p.251.

9.   I. E Harrison, "Traditional Healers: A Neglected Source of Health Manpower" in *African Therapeutic Systems,* p. 198.

10.   Interview with Mr Mafuru, Assistant Chief Nursing Superintendent and Co-ordinator of Primary Health Care, and Mrs E. A. Edemenaha, Senior Nursing Sister in-charge of the Training Programme, Okpe Local Government Council.

11.   P. Berger, "The Precarious Vision, (New York: Doubleday, 1961), p.10 & 11. G.O. Ehusani also used this terminology when he discussed the need for the world to shift from Western Materialistic Cosmology to the African Humanistic Cosmology in *Afro-Christian Vision* (Ibadan: Ambassador Publication, 1972), p.241.

Bibliography

BOOKS

Abraham, W.E. *The Mind of Africa.* Chicago: Chicago Press, 1962.

Achebe, C.C. *The World of the Ogbanje.* Enugu: Fourth Dimension, 1986.

Adesu, M.O. *Understanding African Traditional Religion.* Part One, Sherborne: Dorset Publishing Co., 1985.

Adegbola, A.A. *Traditional Religion in West Africa.* Ibadan: Daystar, 1983.

Ademuwagun, Z.A. et. al. (eds.) *African Therapeutic Systems.* Massachusetts: Crossroads Press, 1979.

Afigbo, A. *Ropes of Sand: Studies in Igbo History and Culture.* Oxford: O.U.P. 1981.

Alland, A. (Jnr.) *Adaptation in Cultural Evolution. An Approach to Medical Anthropology* (NewYork: Columbia University Press, 1970).

Amadi, E. *The Concubine.* Ibadan: Heinemann, 1988.

Andersen, U.S. *Three Magic Words.* California: Wilshire Book Co., 1954.

Arinze, F.A. *Sacrifice in Ibo Religion.* Ibadan: Ibadan University Press, 1970.

Awolalu J.O. *Yoruba Belief and Sacrificial Rites.* London: Longman, 1981.

Awolalu J.O. & Dopamu P.A. *West African Traditional Religion.* Ibadan: Onibonoje Press, 1979.

Awolowo O. *The Peoples Republic.* Ibadan: Heinemann, 1968.

Azikiwe N. *Renascent Africa:* London: Frank Cass, 1968.

Baete C. G. *Prophetism in Ghana: A Study of Some Spiritual Churches.* (London: S.C.M. 1962).

Balogun I.A. Dopamu P.A. et. al. *Place of Religion in the Development of Nigeria,* Ilorin: Dept. of Religion, Unilorin, 1988.

Barbot J. *A Collection of Voyages and Travels.* Vol. 5. London: Maffiurs Churchill, 1946.

Barrets D. B.   *Schism and Renewal in Africa.* Nairobi: O.U.P., 1968.

Bascom W. R.   *The Yoruba of South West Nigeria,* (Holt: Rinehart and Winston, 1969).

Benedict R.   *Patterns of Culture.* London: Routledge & Kegan Paul, 1961.

Bibeau G. et. al. *Traditional Medicine in Zaire: Present and Potential Contribution to the Health Service.*

Bogdon R. & Taylor S.J. *Introduction to Qualitative Research Methods: Phenomenological Approach to Social Sciences.* New York: John Wilney Co., 1975.

Bohan P. & Curtin P. Africa and Africans; (Revised edition). New York: The Natural History Press, 1971.

Booth N.S. (Jnr.) (ed.) *African Religions: A Symposium.* New York: NOK, 1977.

Bosman W.   *A New Account and Accounts Description of the Coast of Guinea.* Blantyre: 1970.

Bozeman A. B. *Conflict in Africa. Concepts and Realities.* New Jersey: Princeton University Press: 1976.

Bradbury R. E.   *The Benin Kingdom and the Edo-speaking Peoples of South Western Nigeria.* London: Wightman Mountain, 1970.

Brockington F. *World Health.* Harmondsworth, Middlesex: Penguin Books, 1958.

Burns A. C.   *History of Nigeria.* New York: Barnes and Nobles, 1944 Reprinted.

Burton, R. F.   *A Mission to King of Dahomey, Vol.* 11. London: Tinsley Brothers, 2nd Edition, 1964.

Busia, K.A.   *The Challenge of Africa.* New York: Frederick A. Praeger, 1962.

Dubois, W.E.B. *The Souls of Black Folks.* Greenwich: Fawcett, 1961.

The World and Africa. Cambridge & Massachusetts: O.U.P., 1962.

Durkheim, E. *The Elementary Forms of the Religious Life.* London: George Allen & Unwin, 1957.

Efenakpo, R.O. *The Ogor Kingdom: A Pictoral History of A People (Ovie Adjara 111. Coronation Souvenir).* Warri: Refe Holding Publishers, 1987.

Egharevba, J.U. *A Short History of Benin.* Ibadan: Ibadan University Press, 1960.

Ehusani, G.O. *An Afro-Christian Vision: Ozovehe.* Ibadan: Ambassador Publications, 1992.

Ejisafe, A.E. *The Laws and Customs of the Yoruba People.* Abeokuta: M.A. Ola & Fola Bookshops, n.d.

Ejizu, C.L *Ofo: Igbo Ritual Symbol.* Enugu: Fourth Dimension Publishing Co, 1986.

Ekpunobi, E.& Ezeaku, I. (eds). *Socio-Philosophical Perspective of African Traditional Religion.* Enugu: New Age Publisher, 1990.

Eliade, M. (ed) *Symbolism, The Sacred and The Arts.* New York: Biane Apostolos-Cappadona Crossroad, 1986.

Ellis, A.B. *The Yoruba-Speaking People of the Slave Coast: Their Religion and Customs,* (London: 1894).

Emekpe, J.L *The History of the Ughelli People of Urhobo Tribe,* (Warri: Kagho Industrial Ltd. 1981.

Erivwo, S.U. *A History of Christianity in Nigeria: The Urhobo, The Isoko and The Itsekiri.* Ibadan: Daystar Press, 1979.

— — — *Traditional Religion and Christianity in Nigeria: The Urhobo People,* Ekpoma: Dept. of Religion & Philosophy, Bendel State University, 1991.

Evans-Pritchard, E. E. *The Theories of Primitive Religion, (Oxford: Clarendon Press, 1965. Nuer Religion.* London: O.U.P., 1970.

Witchcraft, Oracle and Magic Among the Azande. Oxford: Clarendon Press, 1976.

Ezeabasili, N. *African Science: Myth or Reality.* New York: Vantage Press, 1977.

Fajana, A. & Biggs, B.J. Nigeria in History. Ibadan: Longman, 1964.

Fanon, F. *The Wretched of the Earth.* France: Francois Maspero Editeur, 1961.

Field, M.J. *Religion and Medicine of the Ga- People.* London: O.U.P. Reprinted, 1969.

Forde, D. & Jones, G.I. *The Ibo and Ibibio-Speaking People of South Eastern Nigeria,* London: International African Institute, 1950.

Fortes,& Dieter, (eds.) *African System of Thought.* Norwich: O.U.P., 1972.

Friedland, W.& Roseburg, C (eds), *African Socialism.* Standford: S.U.P., 1967.

Frobenius, L.   *The Voice of Africa.* Vol. 1, London: O.U.P., 1913.

Gelfand, M.   *Medicine and Custom in Africa.* Edinburgh & London: E. S. Livingstone, 1964).

   The African Witch. Edinburgh & London: E.S. Livingstone. 1967.

Gennep, A. Van. *The Rites of Passage.* London: Routhledge and Kegan Paul, 1976.

Gheddo, P.   *Why is the Third World Poor?* New York: Orbis Books, 1973

Green, M. M.   *Igbo Village Affairs.* London: Frank Cass, 2nd Edition, 1964.

Guest, G.   *The March of Civilization.* London: G. Bell & Sons, 1961.

Gyekye, Kwame. *An Essay on African Philosophical Thought.* New York: Cambridge University Press, 1987.

Hamdum, S. & King, N. *Ibn Battuta in Black Africa.* London: Rex Collins, 1976.

Harley, G. W.   *Native African Medicine with Special Reference to its Practice in Mano Tribe of Liberia.* London: Frank Cass, 1970.

Harrison, I. E., & Dunlop, D. W. *Traditional Healers Use and Non-Use in Health Care Delivery.* Michigan: Michigan State University, 1974.

Hegel.   *The Philosophy of History.* New York: Dover, 1956.

Hetzel, B. S. (ed.) *Basic Health Care in Developing Countries,* (Oxford: O.U.P., 1978).

Hinschberg.   *Monuments: Ethnographic BD I.* Schwartz-Africa: Gratz/Austrica, 1962.

Hubbard, J.W. *The Sobo of Niger Delta.* Zaria: Gaskiya Corporations, 1948.

Ifemesia, C.   Issues in Africa Studies and National Education, Selected Works of Kenneth Dike, 1978.

....   *Traditional Humane Living among the Igbo: An Historical Perspective.* Enugu: Fourth Dimension, 1979.

Idowu, E. B.   *African Traditional Religion: A Definition.* London: S.C.M. 1973.

....   *Olodumare: God in Yoruba Belief.* Therford: Lane and Brudone, 1977.

Ikime, O.   *Niger Delta Rivalry.* London: Longman, 1974.

Ilogu, E.   *Christianity and Igbo Culture.* London: NOK Publishers, 1974.

Irhueh, A.O. *Image of God in Man.* Rome: Urbaniana University Press, 1987.

Isichei, E. *Igbo Worlds: An Anthology of Oral History and Historical Descriptions.* Philadelphia: Institute of the Study of Human Issues, 1978.

Iwu, M.M. *Traditional Igbo Medicine, Report of a Project Sponsored by the Institute of African Studies, U.N.N., 1981.*

Jackson, The Role of Faith in the Process of Healing. London: S.C.M., 1981.

Jahann, J., *Muntu: An Outline of the New African Culture.* New York: Grove Press, 1961.

Jellife, D.B., (ed) *Child Health in the Tropics.* Washington: Pan American Health Organization, 1979.

Kalu, O.U.(ed). Readings in African Humanities: African Cultural Development, Enugu: Fourth Dimension, 1978.

Kaunda, K.& Moris Collin, (eds.). *A Humanist in African.* Nashville: Abingdon Press, 1966.

Kingsley M. N. *West African Studies.* 3rd Edition, London: Frank Cass & Co., 1964.

Kokwaro J. O, *Medicinal Plants in East African.* Nairobi: East African Literature Bureau, 1976.

Kwesi, D. et. al. (eds.). *Biblical Revelation and African Belief.* London: Lutherwork, 1972.

Lamb, E. *The Africans: Encounter from Sudan to the Cape.* London: 1986.

Lambo, T.A. (ed.). First Pan-African Psychiatric Conference. Abeokuta: Government. Press, 1962.

Last, M.& Chavunduka, G.E. (eds.). *Professionalization of African Medicine.* Manchester: M.U.P., 1986.

Leonard, A.G., *Lower Niger and Its Tribes.* London: 1966.

Levin, A. (ed). *Health Services: The Local Perspective.* New York: Capital City Press, 1977.

Livingstone, W.P. *Dr. Hitchcock of Ubunu: An Episode in Pioneer Missionary Work in Nigeria.* Edinburgh: United Free Church of Scotland Press, 1920.

Maclean, Una, *Magical Medicine: A Nigerian Case Study.* London: Reading and Fakenham, 1971.

Mbefo, L.   *Towards A Mature African Christianity.* Enugu: Fourth Dimension, 1989.

Mbiti, J.S.   *African Religions and Philosophy.* London: Heinemann, 1969.

———   *The Prayers of African Religion.* London: SPCK, 1970.

———   *Introduction to African Religions and Philosophy.* London: Heinemann, 1975.

Mead, M.   *Culture, Health and Disease.* London: Tavistock Publication, 1966.

Metuh, E.I.   *God and Man in African Religion.* London : Geoffrey Chapman, 1981.

———   *The Gods in Retreat: Continuity and Change in African Religions.* Enugu, Fourth Dimension, 1985.

Comparative Studies of African Traditional Religions. Onitsha: Imko, 1987.

Mume, J.O.   *Traditional Medicine in Nigeria.* Agbarho: Jom Nature Cure Centre, n.d.

Tradomedicalism: What It Is? (Agbarho: Jom Nature Cure Centre, n.d.

A Message for All Who Seek Health. Agbarho: Jom Nature Cure Centre, 1973.

Munonye, J. *Obi.* (London: Heinemann, 1976.

Mouroux, J. *The Meaning of Man.* New York: Sheed and Ward, 1948.

Nadel, F. *Nupe Religion.* London: Routledge and Kegan Paul, 1954.

Nwoga, D. *The Supreme God as Stranger in Igbo Religious Thought.* Mbaise: Hawk Press, 1984.

Nwosu, V.A. (ed). *Prayer Houses and Faith Healing.* Onitsha: Tahari Press, 1971.

Nyang, Sulayman *Islam, Christianity and African Identity.* Vermont: 1984.

Okpewho, L. *The Victim.* Ikeja: Longman Drumbeat, 1979.

Okumagba, M.P. *The Short History of the Urhobo.* Nigeria; Kris & Praty n.d.

Oliver, B. *Medicinal Plants in Nigeria.* Ibadan: Nigeria College of Arts and Science, 1960.

Opoku, K.A. *West African Traditional Religion.* Accra: F.E.P. International, 1978.

Otite, O. *Autonomy and Dependence.* Ibadan: Ibadan University Press, 1973.

—— — (ed). *The Urhobo People.* Ibadan: Heinemann, 1982.

Ottenberg, S.& Óttenberg, P. (eds). *Culture and Societies in Africa.* New York: Random Press, 1960.

Parrinder, E.G. *West Africa Religion.* London: Epworth Press, 1969.

—— — *African Traditional Religion.* London: S.C.M., 1969.

Parry, E.H.O. *Principles of Medicine in Africa.* Oxford: O.U.P., 1976.

Pawson, I.G. *Physical Anthropology: Human Evolution.* New York: John Wiley and Sons, 1977.

Payer, L, *Medicine and Culture.* New York: Penguin Books, 1988.

Rattray, R.S. *Ashanti.* Oxford: Clarendon Press, 1923.

—— — Religion and Art in Ashanti. London: 1927.

Ray, B. *Africa Religions: Symbol, Ritual and Community.* New Jersey: Prentice - Hall, 1976.

Reemaeker, *The Philosophy of Being: A Synthesis of Metaphysics,* (London: Herder Book, 1966).

Reth, Hing H. *Great Benin: Its Customs, Art and Horrors.* Halifax &England: F. Kings and Sons, 1902.

Rodney, W. *How Europe Underdeveloped Africa.* Da Es Salam: Tanzania, 1972.

Simpson, G.E. *Yoruba Religion and Medicine in Ibadan.* Ibadan: Ibadan University Press, 1980.

Schneller, P.L. *A Handbook on Inculturation.* New York: Paulist Press, 1990.

Shorter, A. *Africa Culture and the Christian Church.* London : Geoffrey Chapman, 1973.

—— — *Africa Christian Theology: Adaptation or Incarnation?* London: Geoffrey Chapman, 1975.

Smith A. *A Contribution to South African Materia Medica.* Lovedale: South Africa, 1988.

Smurl J. F. *Religious Ethics: A system Approach.* New Jersey: Prentice - Hill, 1972.

Sofowora A. *Medicinal Plants and Traditional Medicine in Africa.* Ibadan : Spectrum

Books, 1984.

Soyinka, Wole. *Idanre and Other Poems.* London: Eyre Mathuen, 1967.

Talbot, P.A. *The Peoples of Southern Nigeria Vol. 11.* London: Frank Cass, 1969.

Taylor, J.V. *The Primal Vision.* London: S.C.M., 1969.

Tempel, P. *Bantu Philosophy.* Paris: Presence Africaine, 1959.

Thiong'O Ngugi Wa. *Writers in Politics.* London: Heinemann, 1981.

——— *Decolonizing the Mind.* London: London University Press, 1986.

Turner, V.W. *The Forest of Symbols.* London: Connell University Press, 1967.

Uchendu, V.C. *The Igbo of South East of Nigeria.* New York: Holt, Rinework and Winston, 1965.

Wells, L.G. *Health, Healing and Society.* Johannesburg: Ravan Press, 1974.

Weiss M. L, & Man, A. E. *Human Biology and Behaviour: An Anthropological Perspective.* Boston & Toronto: Little Brown & Co., 1978.

JOURNAL, ARTICLES AND SEMINAR PAPERS

Aagaard J. "The Cosmology behind Healing Techniques" *Journal of Mission Theology,* Vol. 1, Fasc. 1, 1991.

Ackerman S. E. "The Language of Religious Innovation: Spirit Possession and Exorcism in a Malaysian Catholic Pentecostal Movement", *Journal of Anthropological Research,* Vol. 37, 1981.

Agbedahu J. M. "Religion and Traditional Medicine in Nigeria: The Yoruba Experience", A Paper Presented at the Workshop Organized by the Dept. of Religion, University of Ife, Ile-Ife, June 5-7, 1986.

Animalu A. O. E. "Science, Religion and African Culture" being a Lecture Delivered in a Seminar Organized by the Academy of Science at the Nigerian Institute of International Affairs, Victoria Island, Lagos, 8th April, 1989.

Back C., Martin Luther. "On Sickness and Healing" in *Journal of Mission Theology.* Vol. 1, Fasc. 1, 1991.

Bascom W. R. "Ifa Divination: Communication between God and Man" *West Africa.*

Bloomington: Indiana University Press, 1969.

Berentsen, Jean-Martin. "Opening Address to a Seminar on Healing Ministry" *Journal of Mission.* Vol.1, Fasc. 1, 1991.

Boston J. "Medicine and Fetishes in Igala" *Africa.* Vol. 41, 1972.

Bujo B. "Can Morality be Christian in African?" *African Christian Studies.* Nairobi: March, 1988.

Byaruhanga-Akikiki A. B. T. "Theology of Medicine" *Journey of African Religion.* Vol. 2, No. 1, 1991.

Dopamu P. A. "Yoruba Magic and Medicine and Their Relevance for Today". *RELIGION (NASR)* Vol. 4, Dec. 1979.

Dopamu P. A. "The Secret of Total-Well-Being with Particular Reference to African Religion," *JARS,* (Journal of Arabic and Religious Studies), Vol. 1, Dec. 1984.

Dopamu P. A. "Health and Healing within the Traditional African Religious Contexts". *ORITA* Vol. 17, No. 2 Dec. 1985.

Dopamu P. A. "The Reality of Isasi, Apeta, Ironsi, and Efun as Force of Evil in *JARS,* Vol. 5, 1990.

Echeruo M. J. C. "A Matter of Identity". 1979 Ahiajoku Lectures, Culture Division, Ministry of Information, Culture, Youth and Sports, Owerri.

Ekwunife A. "Consecration in Igbo Traditional Religion", A Thesis Proposal for the Degree of Doctor of Philosophy in Religion, University of Nigeria. Nsukka: 1984.

Ejizu C. I. "Healing as Wholeness: The Igbo Experience" *Africana Marburgeosia* (ed.) by I.T. Hachett Vol. 129. 1988.

Elemi M. E. E. "The Church's Healing Ministry in the Light of African Understanding of Health and Healing". A Term Paper Presented to the Department of Religious Studies and Philosophy Graduate Programme, University of Calabar, March, 1990.

Enang K. "Some Key Religious Concepts of the Anang" *Africana Marburgensia.* (ed. by) R.I.J. Kachett Sonderheft 12: Special Issue 12, 1987.

Engelsviken T. "Exorcism and Healing in the Evangelical Churches of Ethiopia". *Journal of Mission Theology,* Vol.1, Fasc.1, 1991.

Epelle E. M. T. "Development of Sects in Eastern Nigeria" *WAR.* Vol. 14, 1972.

Erivwo S.U. Epha: "Divination System among Urhobo of Niger Delta" *African Notes.* Vol. 8, No. 1, 1979.

Erivwo S.U. "Religion and Identity: The Church's Role in Nation Building with Special Reference to Nigeria". *NASR,* (1988).

Ezeanya, S. N. "Healing in Traditional African Society" *WAR.* Vol. 17, N0.1, 1978.

Forsberg J. "Redemption as Healing, An Ignored Aspect of the Lutheran Tradition", *Journal of Mission Theology.* Vol. 1, Fasc. 1, 1991.

Foster G. M. "Disease Etiologies in Non-Western Medical Systems", *American Anthropologist.* No.78 (1976).

Goodchild J Mck. "Biblical Theology and the Healing Ministry", *WAR.* Vol.17, No. 1, 1976.

Harjula D. R. "The Human Struggle with Guilt". An anthropological Case Study with Some Theological Reflections in *Journal of Mission Theology.* Vol. 1, Fasc. 1, 1991.

Henrisson Carl-Gustav, "Spirituality and Addiction in Northern Tanzania". *Journal of Mission Theology.* Vol. 1, Fasc. 1, 1991.

Hirvonen L. "Healing, Culture and the Concept of Human", *Journal of Mission Theology.* Vol. 1, Fasc. 1, 1991.

Horton R. "African Traditional Thought and Western Science", *AFRICAN.* Vol. 37, Nos. 1 & 2, April 1967.

Ifesieh E.I. "The Concept of Chineke as Reflected in Igbo Names and Proverbs" . *Communio Viatorum,* No. 26, (1983).

Iwu M. M. "Symbolism and Selectivity in Traditional African Medicine". A Lecture Delivered by the Winner of Vice-Chancellor's Research Leadership Prize for 1987, U.N. Nsukka, January 12, 1989.

Iwuagwu A. O. (Rt. Rev.) "The Healing Ministry in the Church in Nigeria" *WAR,* Vol. 17, No. 1, (1976).

Jedrej M. C. "Medicine, Fetish and Secret Society in a West African Culture" *AFRICA,* Vol. 46, 1976.

Juntunen S. "The Holistic Healing by the Charismatic Today in Practice in an Evangelical Lutheran Congregation in Helsinki". *Journal of Mission Theology,* Vol. 1, Fasc. 1, 1991.

Kalu O. U. "An Alive Universe: The African World Over a Century's Presence of the Church in Africa: A Historical Analysis of the Evangelization Process."

Kalu O. U. "Religion, Medicine and Healing in Nigeria." A keynote review at the Third Annual Workshop Organized by the Department of Religion, University of Ife, Ile-Ife (n.d.).

Lande A. "Healing in the New Religions of Japan", in *Journal of Mission Theology.* Vol. 1, Fasc. 1, 1991.

Lartey E. Y. "Healing Traditional and Pentecostalism in Africa Today" *International Review of Mission,* Vol. 74, No.297, Jan. 1986.

Long G. M., "Prolegomenon to a Religious Hermeneutic" *History of Religion,* Vol. 6, No.3, (1971).

Metuh, E. I. "African Traditional Medicine and Healing. A Theological and Pastoral Reappraisal", *LUCERNA,* Jan.- June 1985.

Mume, J. O. "A Traditional Doctor Speaks" *World Health: The Magazine of the World Health Organization,* Oct. 1976.

Nduka O. "Rationality and Technological Development." A Paper Presented at the Silver Jubilee of the Department of Philosophy, University of Nigeria, Nsukka, 1990.

Nkpong, J. "Contextualizing Theological Education in West African", *African Christian Studies:* Nairobi: September 1989.

Nze, C. "Logic in African Charm Medicine", in *The Nigerian Journal of Social Studies: Vol. 4, No.1, (1987).*

Oguakwa, J.U. "Authenticity of African Traditional Medicine Validity and Provocative Consequences: A New Philosophical Dimension in Traditional Medicine". A Paper Presented at the International Workshop on African Philosophy, University of Nigerian, Nsukka, Dec. 13-16, 1990.

Ohiaeri, A.E. "Research in the Traditional Nigerian Medicine", Medical Centre, University of Nigeria, Nsukka (nd).

Omuabor, V. "Face to Face with Juju men", *African Concord. Vol. 38, April 1987.*

Onunwa, U.R. (Rev.) "Psychiatric Care of Traditional Mental". A Paper Presented at the Workshop on Role of Religion, Department of Religion, University of

Ife: 1986.

Osedebe, P.O. "The Independence Movement in Sierra Leone", *TARIK:* Vol. 4, No. 1, 1971.

Osisiogu, L.U.W. "Some Notes on African's Drug Plant Heritage", IKENGA: Vol. 1 No. 2, No 1, 1971.

Otite, O.   "History as a Process: A Study of the Urhobo of the Midwestern State of Nigeria", African Historical Studies, Vol. 4, No. 1, 1971.

Press, I.   Urban Illness: Physician, Cure, and Dual Use of Bogata", Journal of Health and Social Behaviour. No.10, 1969.

Prince, R.,   "The Yoruba Image of the Witch" Journal of Mental Science, No. 107, 1961.

Prince, R.   "Some Notes on Yoruba, Native Doctors and their Management of Mental Illness", Conference Report, First Pan-African Psychiatric *Conference, Abeokuta, Nigerian, 1962.*

Schwartz, L.R.   "The Hierarchy of Resort in Curative Practice: The Admirality Islands, Malanesia", Journal of Health and Social Behaviour. Vol. 10, 1969.

Serkkola, A. "Therapeutic Functions of Islamic Healing in Southern Somalia", Journal of Mission Theology, Vol. 1, Fasc. 1,1991.

Turner, V.W.   "The Way Forward in the Study of Primal Religion", *JRA*, Vol. 3, No. 1, 1981.

Twumasi, P. A. "Scientific Medicine: The Ghanaian Experience", *International Journal of Nursing.* No. 9, 1972.

Ubrurhe, J.O. "Man and the Concept of Hereafter in African Belief System" *AJRS* (Abraka Journal of Religious Studies), Vol. 1, No.1, July 1991.

Uju,J. "Ritual and Symbol in Agwu-Cultic Initiations Among the Igbo". A Paper Presented at the Third Annual Workshop on Igbo Life and Culture Organized by the Institute of African Studies in Association with the Faculty of Arts, U.N.N., Dec. 3-6,1989.

Umude, J.K. The Origin of the Urhobo People: A Critical Look at the Benin Theory", ETA, an Urhobo Cultural Magazine, Magazine, Maiden Issue, 1981.

Uzoma, A.U. The Causal Role of the Word (Okwu) in Igbo Traditional Medicine, A

Paper Presented at the Third Annual Seminar in Igbo Life and Culture organized by Institute of African Studies in Association with the Faculty of Arts, U.N.N., Dec.3-6, 1989.

Ward E., The Yoruba Husband-Wife Code", Anthropological Series, No.6, Washington, D.C: Catholic University of America, 1938.

Wilson, M., Nyakausa, "Ritual and Symbolism", American Anthropologists, Vol. 56, No.2 1954.

Wyllie, R.W. Ghanaian Spiritual and Traditional Healers Explanation of illness: A Preliminary Survey" Journal of Religion. Vol. 14 (1983).

Yamamoto, W.J. Healing and Exorcism in Japanese Folk Religion," Journal of Mission Theology. Vol.1, Fasc.1, 1991.

ENCYCLOPAEDIAS AND DICTIONARIES

Could, J. (ed)   The Dictionary of Social Sciences. Tovistock Publisher, 1964.

Coyne, B. et. al. (eds), The Encyclopaedia Americana International. Connecticut: American Corporation, 1979.

Hastings, J. (ed), Encyclopaedia of Religion and Ethics. Edinburgh: T.& T. Clark, 1971.

Moris, W. (ed), The American Heritage Dictionary of English Language. Boston: Hought of Miffin, 1982.

Onions, C.T. (ed), The Shorter Oxford English Dictionary. Vol. 11, London: O.U.P., 1973.

Sills, D.C. International Encyclopaedia of Social Sciences. Vols. 5 & 6. New York: Macmillan and Free Press, 1972.

UNPUBLISHED THESES AND DISSERTATIONS

Anizoba, O.M. The Dignity of Man in Igbo Traditional Religious Belief, Ph.D. Thesis, Department of Religion, U.N.N., 1986.

Anorue, E.J.C. Problems and Challenges of Healing Churches in Mbano Local Government Area, Master Dissertation, Department of Religion, U.N.N., 1987.

Esiri, P. Witchcraft in Urhobo, B.A. (ed) Dissertation, Department of Religious Studies,

Bendel State University, Abraka Campus, 1988.

Ezea, S.O.K. The Pre-Christian Belief in and Cult of the Supreme Being in Anambra and Imo States of Nigeria, M.A. Dissertation Department of University of Nigeria, Nsukka, 1979.

Ezekwugo, C.U.M. "Chi" in Igbo Religion. Ph.D. Thesis, University of Innerbruck, 1973.

Oluponna, J.O.K. Phenomenological-Anthropological Analysis of Religion of Ondo-Yoruba of Nigeria Ph.D. Thesis, University of Boston, 1983.

Okeke, G.E. The Interpretation of New Testament Teaching on Death and Future Life in African Context. Ph.D. Thesis, Department of Religion, University of Nigeria, Nsukka, 1984.

Onunwa, U.R. The Study of West African Religion in Time Perspective, Ph.D. Thesis, Department of Religion, University of Nigeria Nsukka, 1984.

Nwachukwu, C.C. Religion and Health Care Practice: An Examination of Faith Tabernacle Congregation in Okigwe Local Government Area of Imo State. M.A. Dissertation Proposal, Department of Sociology and Anthropology, University of Nigeria, Nsukka, 1989.

NEWSPAPERS

Traditional Medicine Revisited, *Daily Times,* Aug. 12,1975,

Research in Native Medicine *Daily Times*, Sept. 25,1975.

Federal Ministry of Health, Nigeria, Editorial Comment in Your Health, Vol. 1, No.3, Sept. 1968.

World Health Organization: World Health Directory of Medical Schools, Geneva, 1963.

Problems and Prospects of Trado-Medicine in Nigeria, *Sunday Times,* July 29, 1983.

Integration of Traditional Medicine: Need for Research Caution, *Daily Times,* July19, 1983.

Traditional Healers: Their Roles in Primary Health, *Radio/TV Times*, Nov, 1981.

Curing Infertility in Women: *Sunday Sketch*, February 2, 1986.

Traditional Medicine and National Development: *National Concord*, Monday, February 9,1987.

The Enlarged Prostate in *The Guardian*, Thursday, June 17, 1993.

Mistotle, an example of an all-purpose herb: *The Guardian*, Thursday, June 3, 1993.

The Pains of Impotency and Sterility: *The Guardian*, Thursday, July 22,1993.

Osteoporosis-More in Post Menopausal Women: *The Guardian*, Thursday, July 1,1993.

Women Need Not Have Fibroids: *The Guardian*, Thursday, July 15, 1993.

Disease of the Brain: *The Guardian*, Thursday, July 29,1993.

Why Diseases Recur: *The Guardian*, Thursday, August 5, 1993.

Index